How to Tame Men: a step-by-step Guide to Winning The BATTLE of Sexes

A report by Melanie Raymund

Introduction:

Hi there – my name is Melanie Raymund, and just like you, I struggled to win the man of my dreams. It left me feeling anxious, scared, empty and pretty depressed. However, after YEARS of life-experience and countless hours of research and psychological courses, I cracked the MAN CODE.

It WASN'T easy – but guess what?

I learnt:

- How to make him WANT you like you the single most irresistible human alive
- How to FORCE him to commit, even if he's into multiple women, scared of having his heart broken – or simply isn't into you that much (for now)
- How to almost instantly make a man fall for you on a first date
- How to COMMUNICATE with men and UNDERSTAND men
- How to look at a man and INSTANTLY know if he's into you
- How to KEEP HIM YOURS
- The tale-tale signs that he simply ISN'T and won't EVER be interested in you
- And much MUCH more...

I'm going to cut straight to the chase here...

You want him; you want him bad; and you want him now – but...BUT...you don't know how to get him. You don't know how to stand out of the crowd and win his heart for your own. SO...

In this SPECIAL report, I've put together YEARS of mind-blowing information that will get you that ONE special guy you've always dreamt of having. And what's even better, is that this process is completely achieved in a simple step by step system that is revealed throughout this book.

A word of WARNING though: these techniques are POWERFUL and have been utilised by just a select few women for CENTURIES to great effect.

BUT...before you go ahead and read through the report, you need to PROMISE me that you won't just skim over my proven methods and dismiss them without even trying – OK? These methods work and they work well.

Also – be warned: I don't mess around, so inside the report you will be presented with no fluff, no filler, no BS – nothing but the goods, so that you can finally get the guy you've always wanted – no matter what your situation is.

So, let's great straight into things and start with the reasoning behind...

Why he doesn't want/like you already:

Firstly, let me assume that you REALLY like this guy already – and naturally there comes a certain amount of persistence behind your actions to get what you want in life, correct? You know; the actions that you are already taking to try and make him want/like you back – those actions.

THOSE actions are the ones that are already costing you his heart. Here's an example of what I mean by THOSE actions:

Kelly likes Dan. He's tall, dark, handsome (bla bla bla) – the whole package. And since Kelly likes Dan so much, she texts him every day; she tells her friends how much she likes him; she tells him through text how much she likes him – and she MAYBE even resorts to offering sex in a poor attempt to gain his affection; she dresses up just for him every time they meet up – and makes it extremely obvious that she is into him.

Dan generally likes Kelly, as a friend – but he knows she makes the effort just for him.

Right now, Kelly is YOU (weird if that is already your name). Or she is certainly very similar to you and your situation right now – and here is the problem with persisting in these ways.

What this boils down to is a VERY basic psychological issue amongst most humans, especially men. It is absolutely imbedded into men's nature to want something that they can't have – and if something is offered to them on a nice shiny plate, he will either use that plate (you) for just sex, or completely dismiss there being any chance of having a full blown relationship with you.

So, here are your first steps to take to realign your current relationship with him. This is a short summery, which I will be expanding upon later in the book - so calm down!

- STOP texting him so much – keep your texts short and to the point when you do text.
- DON'T go out of your way just for him. Your life comes before his and he needs to know that.
- DO NOT offer him sex in the hope that it will make him like you more – it won't. A self-respecting female can drive a man insane.
- REMEMBER: this is about making him WANT YOU not making him realise how much you want him.
- DON'T play childish mind-games
- BUT, be prepared to tap into his subconscious mind.

Hey – you wanna know a BIG SECRET, as to what you're probably doing that's pissing up your chances with him? He's some secret sauce for you – and it tastes a lot like bullshit.

You know that guy you 'dig' right now? The one with the body you can fry your breakfast on and the poon-tingling biceps that could crush a goat? The same guy who you are SO desperate to be with that you jump at the chance to get him in bed whenever he likes. The same guy who told you: *'Nah, I'm not looking for anything serious – just some fun'*.

BIG BREATH IN...

The SAME guy who you agreed with and replied: *'Yeh, same here!'*, whilst your brain pinched off a few tears for having to try and sell such a down-right lie, and your entire inner-being dying just a little.

But guess what? That lie – he probably believed it. And now he thinks he has you as his own personal fuck-buddy, and NOTHING more- whilst you hold on to the hope that you could at some point develop a blooming romance through sex alone. Well, you won't – sorry! And that's the harsh truth.

However...DOES HE LIKE YOU ALREADY!?

The reason why you and THAT guy aren't together may sometimes be a non-verbal mutual agreement of shyness between the both of you (in this world, shyness will get you nowhere). So, to find out if the man of your dreams is simply too shy to take the next steps with you – here are a few ways to tell if he currently isn't that into you...

BODY LANGUAGE:

Yeh, yeh – you've heard it all before I'm sure – but believe it or not – body language is actually very telling toward the right eye. The next time you are around him, take a look at which DIRECTION HIS FEET ARE facing. Sound crazy? Well – it's not. The direction of a man's feet can say a lot about his feelings toward you. If his feet are pointing directly toward you, then he feels a subconscious attraction toward you as a person – however, if his feet face away, this usually means he isn't too drawn towards you – YET.

THE EYE OF THE TIGER:

Always keep a look out at what his eyes are telling you. It's a well known fact that a person's pupils will get bigger when talking to you, if they like you. This is of course not an exact science, but it's definitely a factor to look out for!

HELP!

Is your man constantly helping you out with even the smallest of tasks? If so, they he might just be into you. You can do what I call the **'Pencil test'** to see if he is into you. All you need to do is drop a pencil near his feet (not on his feet) and if he is willing to pick it up and then engage in conversation with you afterwards, then it's a good sign – if not, then he's not into you - just yet.

DON'T be scared if these factors are against you at the moment, there is still plenty of time to change the mindset of the male and make him want you more than ever!

THE TIME IS NOW

Now that we've looked over the basics, it's time to get on to the right path and make him want you more than anything on the face of the planet, and even some other planets.

Please be sure to follow each step and don't miss any of the steps out or the whole system will come crashing down!

Ok, sit down, take a big a big breath in, put down your phone, remove Facebook from your life for a couple hours, stop watching 'funny' videos of monkeys eating their own faeces – and ENJOY the rest of the book!

RULE ONE

This is going to take us straight back to the start of the book, but needs to be reiterate to emphasise the importance of this rule – and the first rule is...

DO NOT GIVE YOURSELF TO HIM.

Like I spoke about before, and this is very important: DO NOT give yourself to any man – whether it is for sex or just a casual hang out. A man's brain operates on such a level where he feels that he has to EARN something in his life to truly appreciate it. And if you are handed to him on a silver plate, then he will never fully appreciate you.

So, as I've previously stated; if you find yourself giving in to his every need, then he already knows that there is nothing there for him – he won't value you and therefore will not see you as a viable candidate for a girlfriend.

If it's a case of 'friends with benefits' at the moment, and you're hoping this will lead to something more – it won't. If he begins to approach you for sex again, simply tell him that you're 'BUSY' – this will then trigger one of two emotional responses from him.

DONKEY SHIT

The first reaction is what I call **'The Pattern Breaker'** – and what this does is throw him off guard and breaks down his emotional barriers. Men don't like SUDDEN CHANGE, and if you start changing up his usual expectations, his emotional barriers will start to come right down. What happened when you read the words 'DONKEY SHIT'? You didn't expect it, and it grabbed your attention – same rules apply here!

The second reaction will be an assumption. It's within most men's nature to want to be the ALPHA MALE – thus expecting full well to be bigger and better than every other guy out there. His assumption when you tell him that you're 'BUSY' will almost always make him assume you are getting the goods ELSEWHERE.

Whilst I don't want to turn this book into a 'Play his game' type of book – this alone can be enough to drive a man wild. The thought of being inferior to another male will play on a guys mind for a LONG time – trust me.

So like I said, I don't want to turn the book into something where you are constantly playing games to make him want you – but more so the first step is about CHANGE and changing the rhythm of how things currently are. This will show him you are NOT there for him whenever he requires you and will gain you instant respect.

Not getting what he wants will ALWAYS be a mental stimulator for him; he will see it as a challenge and want to pursue you further.

So let's summarise your first steps:

1. **Don't give into him when he needs you**
2. **Tell him you are 'busy' and leave it at that**
3. **Force him to respect you**

All the above is the FIRST STEP to making a guy want to commit to being with you, and not just using you when he needs.

Remember:

'Donkey Shit'

Now turn the page!

Now let's move on to STEP TWO

RULE TWO

The second rule is all about CHANGE – and changing you.

Now, you may be thinking 'I shouldn't have to change who I am to get this guy' and that's absolutely correct – HOWEVER, the chances are, that you have already CHANGED to be an idea of what you think the perfect girl is.

What it boils down to in 90% of cases, is...**BEING TOO NICE.**

Now, that's not to say that you have to be a complete and utter uber-bitch, but if you are trying to impress your guy by taking the ultra-friendly route, then you are almost certain to fail – and here's why:

Being nice can sometimes come across as 'smothering' – and by being nice you may think that texting him every morning and evening to see how he's doing, is the right thing to do – but it's not. Men enjoy their freedom, and if you continue to act overly-nice, he will look for an escape route in order to help protect what he sees as 'freedom', which will ultimately push him even further away from you.

So...what type of person do you strive to be? A healthier person? A more active person? A person who does things THEY want to do? A person who doesn't get pushed around? A person who lives a care-free life?

Of course these are the things you want to be like; everyone does – and right now, being a slave to the man's needs is you CHANGING from what you naturally want to be, and that's the best person you can be, right?

Once you've taken control over your life, the man will start to REPSECT you more. And given that men LOVE competition, he will start to see you as someone he can start competing for. Looking at someone who loves their own life comes across VERY attractive, not just for men, but women as well.

Your idea of 'nice' may involve deviating from this lifestyle and trying to become the girl YOU THINK he wants you to do. But trust me, FOCUS on YOUR life first before anyone else's and you will start to gain HIS attention and not need to go seeking it.

READ THIS BIT

As previously stated, the idea isn't to CHANGE who you are for him, but to focus on becoming the person you want to be. While that may seem to deviate from your desired path regarding him, it's a must!

You will read in other books that men LOVE bitches – and it's true, we do. But I can assure you that we don't see them as superior relationship candidates. The reason why a lot of men like 'bitches' is because a bitch comes across self-dependant, confident and focused on her own life.

However, what else comes with being a 'bitch'? Selfishness, rudeness, slutty attributes and lots of poor morals. NONE of these things can be considered attractive features in the long-run, can they? The initial attraction to a bitch will be the confidence and independence.

Striving to become a more confident and independent person is what will set you apart from the bitches and make you the desirable person for a long-term relationship.

'Be a prize – and he will compete to win you!' – No idea, but its true!

ALSO...

You also need to take into consideration, that when a man is looking for a viable candidate for a committed relationship, he is studying YOU – and everything about you. If a man can see that there is some emotional baggage attached to you, or some other issue you may have, he WILL find it, and it WILL turn him away from you.

Nobody should have to change for a man – no one. But if there are issues in your life that you may deem 'unattractive' then it is best to resolve them first before moving on with your man.

RULE THREE

Now, let's get down to what a lot of relationships hinge on – and that is...

SEX.

It's already well known that men are more open to sex at an early stage of a relationship than women. Most men will want to have sex first and then gauge from there whether or not the female is worthy enough to be in a relationship. However, this actually gives you a great chance to put the ball firmly in your side of the course – and here's why:

As we touched on earlier, it is human nature to want what you can't have. And not giving into sex at the first chance he gets you alone is only going to make him want you more.

Here is a man's process when it comes to a relationship:

Step one – Sleep with her to see how good she is in bed.

Step two – She can be my girlfriend.

Now, if we completely eliminate the possibility of allowing him to get sex whenever he wants it, you are only then left with the possibility of being his girlfriend in order to get sex with you.

This is somewhat a poor advertisement for the male race, but it's true and it works time and time again. Elimination the option for sex may seem like you will fall into the 'friend zone' as many teenagers will call it – but if you implement the steps in the course to this point, then you will have no problem keeping his attention.

And this works even more so if you man is a 'player' and likes to be involved with multiple women. Whilst it may hurt to think about your man having sex with another woman, you need to ignore it because it is for YOUR benefit that he is doing this. Whilst he can have the most gorgeous girl in his bed whenever he wants, it will be nowhere near as desirable as NOT being able to have it – TRUST ME!

Another great reason to not give into his SEXUAL needs straight away is because of sexual behaviour before and after sex. Let me explain...

Before having sex, a man doesn't know what he wants. His mind is over-run with thoughts of getting the ultimate in all pleasures; it clouds his judgement and might make you come across as the most desirable female alive. However, after sex, the man DOES know what he wants – his mind is clear and he can then form the correct decision for him. Whereas with women, it's the complete opposite.

So if you are giving yourself up to this guy for sex, he will be able to convince you time and time again that he wants you – because he isn't thinking straight. He will move heaven and earth to get into your pants. This isn't always through deceptiveness of course, it's just the nature of a man prior to having sex – he won't know truly what he wants.

In most cases, the female will see sex as 'the spark' and the man will see it as 'just sex'. Creating that spark doesn't come from dropping your knickers the first time he invites you around, the spark comes later – don't ever confuse sex with the spark.

So let's quickly summarise what we know about sex now.

DON'T give it to him when he wants it

DON'T give him the option to be just 'friends with benefits'

ONLY have sex after he's committed to the relationship

IF he wants you – he HAS to commit

Now the next step, I want to talk about HIM.

RULE FOUR

In this chapter, I wanted to talk a little bit more about HIM, not you – and why exactly he may be TOO SCARED to commit and what actions you can take to combat this fear.

The guy you are after may lust you, he may love you, he may adore you from the bottom of his soul – but that doesn't mean he is prepared to commit to being 'yours' – and here are the reasons why:

Reason one – He's been 'burnt' before.

No matter whom he is; how he comes across; what he tells you, he will be EXTREMELY reluctant to commit if he's had his heart broken in the past. Even if he appears to be the alpha male amongst alpha males – this can still be an extreme barrier for lots of men to break through. Nobody likes having their hearts broken – nobody! And as they say: 'Once bitten, twice shy'

The truth of the matter is that if he doesn't jump at the chance to commit to you already, then he could have this problem – and let's be honest, a LOT of people have been through at least one heart break.

The solution

Unfortunately there is no TRUE, 100% solution to this problem. Getting involved with a man who is in need of being 'fixed' is a dangerous position. He won't know truly what he wants – and this could end up backfiring on your entire plan.

In order for a long term relationship to pan out, there has to be absolutely conviction that the other party isn't going to break your heart – without that, you have nothing stable, nothing to be TRULY happy about.

No matter what ANY book tells you; there is NO exact science to getting a guy to want to be with you – especially when it comes to broken hearts. The only thing you can do is to give him a REASON to trust you now – so if the time comes he wants to commit, then he will safer doing so.

Be reliable. Don't fall into the category of being a 'bitch' – but at the same time, don't let him walk over you just because of any hurtful past he may have had. If you plan to hook up for a date with him at some point, make sure you are PROMPT with your timing and never cancel last minute – this is the ultimate trust-breaker. The bitch approach may be to stand him up, or arrive late to the date – and whilst this may make a man want you more, it will definitely do no good for his trust in you.

Remember: give him a REASON to TRUST you.

And be a trustworthy person.

Reason two – loss of his free time

Some guys will be happy to jump straight into a relationship – but if you are reading this book, then chances are that your guy...ain't that type of guy – and one of the biggest reasons why he won't commit to being yours; is that he may be scared of losing his precious free time. You know, the time he has with his buddies, playing video games, playing sports and so on.

The fear of having these things taken away from a man can be crippling to the conscious mind of any male – and as soon as he starts feeling things may be getting too 'serious' between him and you, he will most likely start to back off.

Solution:

The solution is obvious.

LET HIM HAVE WHATEVER TIME HE WANTS.

This applies to whatever your current situation with him is. If you and him are currently 'seeing' each other, then make sure you give him whatever free time he wants – and if he wants to go out with his buddies for the night instead of doing something with you, then LET HIM – and DON'T complain or try to make him change his mind. After all, this is something he WANTS to do.

And if you are allowing your man to do the things he wants to do, then he will almost certainly be more willing to take you up on any 'date' offer you may have with him in the future – which leads to the NEXT STEP in this course of what to do next.

MAKING A MOVE ON HIM

Ok, so now we are going to get into the 'meat' of the book.

It's all very well allowing your man his time, not texting him, not fussing over other women he may be dating – BUT...but where does this actually get you if you don't take some form of action? That's right, nowhere!

Whilst everything in the course is designed to make the man want you more, you still need to let him know that you MIGHT be interested in him – but never fully disclose that.

Here are some steps you should have taken so far:

1. You have stopped your needy and persistent text messages to him.
2. You allow him to get on with his life and don't try to force him to make plans with you especially if he is seeing another woman – you let him do what he wants.
3. You've built up a certain degree of trust between each other (this is important)
4. I didn't discuss this earlier, but if you have problems in your life that you want to complain about – DO IT TO A FRIEND AND NOT HIM.
5. And finally, you are making sure that you are not jumping at the chance to get in bed with him, if this is your current situation, make sure it changes and he knows that he can't have you that easily.

HOWEVER...

There is another step that needs to take place, and that is out of your control – and this is a vital step. But you need to WAIT for him to make some form of contact with you. Whilst I don't want to make this book fall into the category of 'mind playing teenager games' – there is still an element of that required here.

In order for you to take the next step with your guy, there HAS to be some sort of signal coming from him – and no matter what any other book tells you; if he doesn't feel that attraction to you, there may be nothing more you can do. HOWEVER, if you have already fallen into the 'friends with benefits' category, then this is actually a good sign, as it shows there is definitely an attraction there.

But do please bear in mind, that when I say there needs to be some form of attraction, this can be the SLIGHTEST of attractions – and not necessarily a physical one either. A strong and controlled personality can be a VERY attractive trait, even toward shallow men.

Ok, now here are a few common signals that your guy is starting to try and grab your attention and may be interested.

- He starts texting you first
- He starts 'liking' your Facebook posts (yuck)

- He compliments you, instead of instantly trying to bed you
- He starts up conversations with you when you see him
- Most of his attention is on you when you are in groups of friends
- He might try and make you feel jealous about another girl he's seeing
- He sticks rigorously to any plans you make with him
- He asks about you to your friends
- He mentions that he 'works out'
- He will come up with silly reasons to get you and him in the same place alone
- He gets jealous about other guys in your life

A note on jealousy:

A little bit of jealousy is natural, it's fine and it's sometimes needed to know that we are wanted – however, as a lot of these type of 'get the guy' books tell you to do, you should never go overboard with making him feel jealous.

Telling him how 'hot' that new guy you met at the bar last night is, isn't going to do him any good – and bragging about how good another man's penis is, certainly won't help. There will eventually become a point in this sad little mind game so many people decide to play, where the guy will simply feel INADEQUATE and just give up on you.

Making another person feel that jealous is plain WRONG, so don't do it – but feel free to use it in moderation. If you tell him that you are busy with another 'friend' – he will instantly assume that you're going over another guys apartment for sex – trust me, he will assume the worst as soon as you start mentioning other 'friends'. And that is fine, it won't drive him mad, but his imagination will get the better of him eventually.

The main goal with using jealousy to your advantage is to NOT make him feel that your standards are so high that they can't be met by him. It may work in the short run, but if you keep that type of mind-game up with him, you're fucked – and not in the nice way.

Ok, let's continue where we left off...

So you need to make sure that he is starting to show a little bit more interest in you, and not just wanting to get a quick lay down, genuine interest about your day and you as a person. Shall we just call it small talk?

The temptation from here is to simply ask him out on a date. WRONG – don't do it; that gives him all the power he needs again – just like your original situation with him. What needs to happen is...

HE has to be the one to ask YOU out on a date. He needs to at least believe that the idea of you and him getting together is his own idea, not yours. And you can achieve this in certain situations very easily.

If he calls or texts you asking if you want to hang out, deny him the chance of thinking he is instantly going to get sex from you at the end of the night.

SECRET METHOD

This works and absolute treat to making a guy take you out on a date, whilst thinking it's his own idea. And this is best when texting, let me give you an example:

Hot stud: 'Heey gurrrl – wanna hang out tonight?'

You: 'No thanks!'

Hot stud: 'Oh, ok...'

You: 'But if you want to take me out for dinner on Saturday at 8, that's your choice'

Hot stud: 'Ok great! I'd love to take you out'

Ok so this approach doesn't need to be taken word for word, but what is does is offset the mind of the male. He won't be used to you saying 'no' to him – so as soon as he receives messages denying him any chance of seeing you, he will instantly assume you aren't interested. But theeeeeeen, the contrast in feelings of not being able to see, to being able to take you out to dinner, in such a short time, will make him JUMP at the chance to take you out.

PURE RELIEF FOR HIM.

Does that make sense? You are either giving him the option to NOT see you at all – or take you out on a date, which you FORCE him to do – thus making it feel like it's his own idea that the two of you 'date'.

Simple? Simple.

NOW SHOULD I SLEEP WITH HIM?

This is your choice. If after your date with him, you want to go back to his and 'bump uglies', then go ahead. You've already taken yourself out of the fuck buddy zone with him as soon as he asked you out on a date.

However, from experience, it's so much sweeter to make him sweat for it. Again, I need to reiterate that I don't want this book to become about childish mind games – but if you really want to make him crave seeing you again – then don't give him sex after your first date with him.

As soon as you leave him to the rest of his evening with his penis and internet – he's going to start thinking that he didn't impress you enough with the 'date' that you guys just went on. And what happens when he starts to think he didn't do well enough? That's right, he starts to compete (as we already know, men love to compete – it's in their nature).

So, the next step he will most likely try and take, is to ask you out on another date – a proper date, again, since he knows he won't get sex just from inviting you back to his place. And this time; he's going to try and impress you and convince you that he is the best guy on the planet, whilst you become even more desirable to him.

My advice: wait til the FORTH date. Any longer and he's gonna get turned off and think you are as frigid as a duck.

Moving on though, we need to take a quick **REALITY CHECK.**

REALITY CHECK

If you are reading through this book, thanks – but more importantly, if you have got to this point and your guy is still trying to just hook up with you for sex or treats you like shit, then there needs to be a point where you simply...

DITCH HIS ASS.

Sometimes there are just men out there who want to try and screw and screw over as many women as humanly possible. Some men will happily go through life breaking hearts, telling lies and doing what it takes to get between your legs.

These guys are also known as DOUCHE BAGS.

If your man isn't treating you with the respect you deserve, then it's time to move on – don't even bother giving him an ultimatum, because it's quite obvious that the little boy isn't ready to grow up and commit to one person any time soon.

Take a good look at yourself before you let any man treat you this way. You already know you are a fantastic, respectable, strong and independent woman who knows what she wants. Why let a man try and take that away from you?

If you want to be fuck-buddies with him, that's your choice – and isn't what this book is about. In fact, I don't think there will ever be a book made to teach women how to get a man into bed. Well, not one that's more than a sentence long anyway...

Here are a few signs to determine whether your guy is a douche-guy:

- He still uses 'lines' to try and pick you up. 'Lines' are for teenagers...and douchebags.
- He goes out of his way to play 'mind games' with you
- He has more than 2 women on the go at once
- He wants to have unprotected sex with you after your first date or anytime.
- He is ashamed to talk to any of his buddies about you
  Quite frankly, the signs will be VERY obvious that if after following the advice in this course, and he still acts like a douche, that he obviously isn't ready to be anyone's boyfriend.

And if he isn't - then so what? There are millions and millions of men out there who would kill to have you on their arm (and other places). You've already taken a big step in purchasing this book, which shows that you're a determined enough person to do whatever it takes to have the life you deserve. And THAT is the most attractive quality a woman can possess.

Anyway, enough of the feel good factor – let's press on.

Why he SHOULD want you now

Ok, so at the start of the book, we spoke about why he doesn't want to be your boyfriend, and addressed the mistakes you were making. Now, let's make a summary as to why he SHOULD want you now – provided that you can safely say he's not a complete douche.

- You've dropped the needy act (texting, calling, begging etc...)
- You don't drop your pants for him upon request
- You are FORCING him to respect you
- You are becoming a prize in his life that he will seek to win
- You are focusing on bettering YOUR life, not his

- You are playing the jealousy game, WITHIN REASON
- You have forced him to take you out on a date
- You are only letting him have sex with you if he's EARNT it
- When he goes home, he's thinking about YOU

The steps taken in this book are 100% designed to make you are more desirable and attractive person, without taking too many childish routes. However, there is NO exact science to making someone you like your boyfriend. Sometimes after all else has failed, there is nothing left – and he simply isn't interested at all – and that is the HARSH but TRUE reality behind things.

This can be a huge blow to a person's self-esteem, and can leave a girl feeling done for. So, in this part of the book, we will take a look at a few ways that will help you keep your mind off a certain person, enjoy your life – and eventually, you will meet someone special, I can assure you.

Remember: there are millions of men out there for you – missing out on just one really isn't the end of the word.

'You know that person you thought you couldn't live without? Well, here you are – all living and shit!' – Don't know!

I know...

Forgetting about someone that you are so infatuated with can be a hard task – but here are a few suggestions that should keep your mind intact.

Join the gym:

Ok, seems a bit silly, right? But you'd be surprised what joining the gym can do for not only your physical health, but also your mental health. I don't want to get into the exact mechanics of why it's so good for you – but trust me, join a gym and you will start feeling 10 times better about yourself, more confident and stress a whole load less.

If you can't afford to join the gym, or there is one nearby, then I suggest taking up some form of yoga, which can be extremely regarding for mind, body and soul!

Also, the chances of meeting someone will GREATLY improve – and gives you the chance to actually meet someone naturally, and build a new relationship from scratch using the methods in this book.

I don't want people to read this and then put up with the disappointment of being given advice such as 'join a gym' – but trust me, I have recommended this advice to many women who are actively seeking for men, and there will SWEAR by it.

And you never know, you may just meet Hans with the big hands from Germany...

Try it!

Focus on self improvement:

This is huge, and in fact, you can totally change your life and relationships simply by focusing all your efforts on YOUR life.

Strive your best to be the person you want to be, and then others around you will be naturally attracted to you.

Aim toward your goals. What do you want from your career? What do you want to achieve health-wise? Where do you want to be in 6 months time?

And I'm sure you've heard all this 'junk' before – but trust me, self-improvement will change your life as long as you make the effort.

Take a break from worrying!

What does worrying actually achieve? Set aside a time of the week which can be your personal worrying time – and if a man has you worrying THAT much, then he might not be worth the mental struggle.

Worrying will only lead to desperation and desperate measures, which will ultimately only decrease your chances of getting that guy.

Now it's time to reiterate a very important part of this book...

Do NOT play games...

After doing a LOT of research as to what ways women want to get themselves a new man, I found that MOST are not interested in playing childish mind-games. And that's good – because personal experience has taught me many things, and one of those things is that mind-games are pathetic.

Sure, as suggested throughout the book, there are a few tiny, little ways you can get into a man's head to your advantage that won't put him off you. But the temptation is to go full-on with these games and try to make your man fall into your arms through jealously alone.

Don't do it!

Sometimes it's FINE to make your guy sweat a little bit – jealously is natural, but making someone want to feel excessive amounts of it, isn't! So, here are a few things you need to bear in mind, or risk losing your man.

- NEVER brag about how 'hot' another guy is that you've met or slept with
- NEVER ditch him last minute for another guy
- NEVER tell him his penis is too small...(oh boy)
- Do NOT try to make him feel like he's not attractive enough for you
- Feel free to go out on OTHER dates whilst you are seeing him, but never brag about them
- Feel free to use the jealously game in very very moderate amounts – but only subtly.

Just remember, if you decide to take up the mind-games approach, you risk losing everything you've worked for. As I said before, a man's ego is very fragile and if broken, he certainly won't be interested in having it broken by you again.

Ok, the next section of the book is going to focus on what to do when you have him FINALLY committed to a relationship.

MIND GAMES

ARE

FOR

CHILDREN

(and insecure bitches...)

When in a relationship

Ok, so hopefully the time has come where you have finally got your man to commit. Good times! Well, now it's time to make sure that he stays committed and you enjoy hopefully a long-term relationship.

A lot of what we discussed earlier about not being needy applies here too. So, for the sake of not repeating myself too much; here is a list of ways to keep him constantly excited to have your company:

- Give him HIS own time and space. If he wants to play the latest version of Call of Duty (blaaah) on his own, let him – leave him to it. If he wants to go chill with his friends, let him. Now's not the time to try and force him onto dates that should come naturally now you are together!
- Don't sleep with him (what, this again???). Of course, sex is an important part of being in a relationship – but that too can get old. Take a few nights off from letting him have his way with you. It will keep him attracted and keen!
- Be fucking AWESOME! The whole point of a relationship is to ultimately be happy, right? And if you are constantly showing your guy what an awesome person you are, he's bound to keep his interest.
- Continue to make him EARN you – even when you are in a committed relationship
- Leave all jealousy and mind games behind! Now's not the time.
- Keep EMOTIONALLY grounded. Sure it's a good outlet to moan to him about your problems – but keep them brief and don't try and expect him to be the solution.
- Keep going out on dates – BUT...and here comes some very SECRET SAUCE.....

The BEST way to make him fall for you

And here is a little bit of secret sauce to keep you thinking. Want to know the bestest of best ways to make a guy fall for you?

Go out on EXCITING dates – and by exciting I don't mean going to the movies or to your local bar. Try taking your man out somewhere that will get his heart racing, his adrenaline pumping and his mind racing. And why's that you ask?

Because doing exciting things that make you feel adrenaline has it's similarities with the feeling of love. If say you were to take him out to a theme park and you went on a rollercoaster – how does it feel? It's exciting; it makes your heart pound; your adrenaline rises, and you feel good when you finish, right? Well, taking a guy out on an exciting date like that is going to associate those feelings with you, because you were the one sharing them with him.

You don't need to do this EVERY date you go on – but I'd recommend doing something exciting at least twice a month. And don't forget to neglect your nights in together – there are the best way to really 'bond' and develop things with each other.

Love is a crazy thing, and we should never try and force another person to love us. We can however hurry it along a little bit!

And if you achieve love, well done! You will sure as hell want to stay in love once you get there.

Staying in love

Staying in love is something anyone in a serious relationship wants to achieve – but unfortunately, it's easier said than done. But my husband and I have been madly in love for many years now – and it's time for me to reveal our secrets.

Now, I don't want to romanticise things here and tell you the secrets revolve around watching The Titanic together in a candle lit room on top of a Greek mountain. However, there needs to be factors that hold the love together and keep it fresh.

Keep your date ideas fresh. The same concept applies as before when you were casually dating. The more exciting the memories, the more likely each of you will be motivated to keep going. Here are a few activities me and my husband engage in on a monthly basis:

- Going to the gym together (three times a week)
- Visiting different restaurants (one a month)
- Going on holiday together (three times a year)
- Trying something completely outrageously new (who would have thought paintball could hurt so much?!)
- Inventive sex...Not much more needs to be disclosed there. You have internet access don't you?

Now of course that means you should never neglect spending one-on-one time together. There needs to be a fine balance of:

- Trying new date ideas
- Spending one-on-one time together
- And allowing each other your own personal time

Time alone is VITAL. At the beginning of a relationship you will of course want to spend as much time together as possible – but as things start to get more serious, you will get to the point where you want to move your own life forward.

And spending 'you' time is the best way to achieve this. I like to take a couple days out of the week at any given point to 'do my own thing'. And you should allow your man to do the same whenever he feels fit. However, you may be thinking, if you are the paranoid type; 'if I let my man do his own thing, won't he cheat?' This moves us on...

Being Faithful – or not

Whenever you want to admit it or not – the harsh truth is that BOTH men and women can be unfaithful, but the reasons for being unfaithful are not usually the same. In order to keep your man faithful, you need to understand the reasons behind why he may NOT stay faithful.

A quick note first: I know this section is hard to read, and you, like most people, will have the attitude that 'he shouldn't be unfaithful if he loves me' – and that's true, he shouldn't. But men are a completely different beast to women and operate on different levels. I hate having to talk about this, but I wanted this book to be the absolute truth, and provide you with everything you need.

So – why do men cheat?

<u>Because they want out</u> – A lot of people, especially men, simply don't have the courage to step up and end a relationship. Cheating on their partner is an easy way for them to send the message and initiate a quick break-up.

Solution – Again, this boils down to the beef of this book: keeping each other happy. If your man isn't happy with how things are with you, then cheating is a realistic solution for him.

<u>It's in their genes</u> – Evolution of man may have physically changed, but the basic mental wiring of a man is to spread his seed throughout as many women as possible. This reason alone may account for the huge numbers of adultery in men alone.

Solution – Harsh secret sauce here for you that will surely burn – but...there really is no solution here. Either your man is like that because of his genes, or he isn't.

You cheated on him – Now, I'm going to make the assumption that this ISN'T going to be the case and that if you aren't happy in the relationship you will end it with respect and class. However, if a woman chooses to cheat on a man, then she can expect the very same treatment back. Consider it revenge sex.

Solution – Don't cheat.

The sex has gone – Men have a higher sex drive than women. Well, in most cases anyway. Men have an insatiable drive for sex, and if they aren't getting it from one source, they may look for another.

Solution - Do your BEST to keep the sex in your relationship enjoyable. Figure out new ways to please each other. There is nothing more 'connecting' than being able to experiment with your partner sexually. Like I said before: you have the whole internet at your disposal for ideas, so don't be afraid to use it.

P.s – and just because that one website tells you to shove that banana up with ass, doesn't mean you have to try that. Discuss with your partner what THEY like as well as you.

Sexual Trophies – A lot of men love to 'hunt' down sexual trophies. The thrill of changing between women and adding an extra notch to their bedpost can be a game that is hard to leave behind for some men. This doesn't mean that he's bored of you, just that he still hasn't taken the time to grow up and respect women.

Solution – Well, this is something that needs to be determined by you prior to committing to a relationship with him. It's your duty to find out about his past, and do whatever it takes to do so! If your man has a reputation for cheating, or sleeping with an unusual amount of women, then you may want to AVOID before you commit.

From my experience: once a cheat, always a cheat.

Ego booster – Men just LOVE to know that they are sexually desirable – and being in a long term relationship can take its toll on a man's ego. Am I still attractive to women? Do they still find me dead sexy? And what an ego boost it really is for a man to find out he still is. Whether this comes from you or not, is another question.

Solution – Make him feel sexy. That's not to say you have to spread sugar all over his ego every five minutes. But every now and again, remind your man that you want him still, in every way possible. This is one of those situations where it's OK to lie just a little ;)

No more love – Let's get one thing straight. It is EXCEPTIONALLY rare for loving relationships to last forever – and let's be honest; nothing last forever. NOTHING. And if your man gets to that point where he simply doesn't love you anymore, then he may not leave you, but he may just turn elsewhere for sexual gratification.

Relationships are hard to break from, even if the love isn't there anymore. The thought of ending something that has been built up for months and maybe years, may seem inconceivable – and there is a good chance that if he doesn't love you, he will stay with you but get his sexual 'fix' elsewhere.

Solution – Usually when the love 'goes' from a relationship, it's easy to start seeing the signs. The two of you may become slightly more distant – and as soon as you get to that point, you need to have a 'chat' with your man.

The worst thing you can do is prolong the experience and hope that the two of you will start seeing sparks again. If things aren't meant to be in the long, long-run, then it most likely won't happen.

Your best bet may be to take some 'time apart' and then get together for some dates and see if you miss being in each other's life's. If you find that the spark doesn't reappear, then it may be a safe bet to try and stay friends.

Losing love in your life is hard, and you should strive to keep it. Be a fun and loving person and love will stay in your life for many years.

I'm sorry if this section isn't what you want to hear, but it's the absolute truth. Holding onto something that isn't there is only going to waste precious moments of your life. There will always be another person out there for you.

And what a lot of staying in love boils down to, is...

Communication

But more specifically: communication with men.

Ok I got a looooot of emails asking me about communication with men. And it seems like a lot of these 'books' don't have this type of info – so let's do this.

He means what he says (for the most part)

Ok so listen up, men operate on a completely different level of communication than women. In fact, men are a LOT more literal in their words than women.

For the most part, men say what the mean – there are no hidden codes or secret emotions hidden in their responses. Unlike women, who tend to hide a lot in their communications, expecting the man to pick up on them.

This is where a lot of communication in relationships break down. One gender plays it one way, and the other plays it the other way. Men are mostly simple-minded and tell things how they are. So when he says something, take it the way it's been said and don't look for a deeper meaning, as there most likely isn't one.

At the same time, don't operate like a typical female in this situation; don't hide your emotions in code-like messages for him to deceiver, because chances are that he will take it as it sounds! Example: don't tell him your 'fine' if you really aren't! He will leave it at that and nothing will get solved.

Emotional wiring

Men and women are wired differently when it comes to emotions. A woman's emotions can go very deep and complex – whereas a man's emotions may not range too far from simply being 'happy', 'sad' or 'angry'. This can become massively confusing and frustrating when it comes to trying to communicate with your man.

While you might be hassling him to find out a more complex reason to his current emotion, he simply may not be able to give you one. Never try to pry open your man's emotions, because unlike us, there is not much more than meets the eye!

Accept what he tells you in terms of how he's currently feeling. If he tells you he feels sad, don't pry and try to find the source. Simply tell him you are there for him if he needs.

If you continue to do so, it will only make him frustrated and tired of you.

Arguments

Arguments – if you're not having any of these whatsoever then something is wrong! They are a natural part of being in a relationship and correct communication is vital when they occur.

Arguments escalate to the point of break ups for one reason – and that is a lack of understanding. As I said before, men and women are 'wired' differently when it comes to approaching things like this.

Let's take a look at a typical argument between genders.

Female: *'Why can't we see each other more often?!'*

Male: '*Because I'm busy with work a lot*'

Female: '*Why can't you take time off work?!*'

Male: '*I can't afford to*'

Female: '*Why can't you afford to? You earn more than me don't?*'

Male: '*I've got rent to pay*'

Etc etc..

The above is an example of the difference in communication when arguing. Whilst it's in a man's NATURE and GENES to want to resolve issues as bluntly and quickly as possible, women act different, as you well know. A woman, when arguing, is looking to 'collect data' and gather as much information as possible whilst finding the very route of every single issue.

Now, what happens when these two styles collide? **KABOOM!**

A tiny tiff can lead to a heated argument and irrational decisions within minutes when these two styles collide.

The problem when arguing with a man and having to put up with his direct responses, is that we ALWAYS assume he is trying to wind us up on purchase; trying to make us angry – but the truth is that he wants to resolve the issue just as much as we do. He just has a different way of approaching it.

So, whenever you argue next, bear this in mind, and try and take things down to his level and don't probe too much, or you will end up hitting the roof and none the wiser.

Compliments

Everyone likes a compliment, right? Right! But your man doesn't seem to be dishing them out to you – why?

Again. Simple. From a younger age, females are taught to dish out compliments – and use compliments are a successful way to communicate with another person and build 'bonds' – call it instincts. While we may dish out compliments, it may not be exactly what is on our minds. However...

Media has hit our generation and gender - and its hit HARD. Beauty magazines tend to focus primarily on what a women's image 'should' look like, and their idea of what attractive is. We've all seen those magazines with the ultra skinny bitches that could fit between the gaps in your front teeth.

And this 'image' is constantly drilled into our minds as to what a 'healthy' and 'attractive' look is. So, naturally, we are overly critical of our look – and to deflect the possibility of receiving potential criticism, we dish out a LOT of compliments. Make sense?

But isn't it just pissy when you don't receive them back? Especially from the guy you like/are with.

Men are again different in this category. Men HAVEN'T been raised to compliment others. Men DON'T have to put up with the constant strain of mainstream media. Sure, there are a lot of male models plastered around magazines grabbing their junk – but the pressure is much, much less to look 'good'.

So whilst men do LIKE compliments, they don't actively seek them in order to feel secure. And what's the best way to get compliments? That's right, by giving them!

Time for me to SHUT UP and present to you the next section of this book:

THE ART OF TEXTING: HOW TO TEXT MEN

Hello there! My name is Melanie Raymund. It's a pleasure to meet you and thanks for taking a look at my report!

I made this report purely from request alone.

Whether we like it or not – texting is now a HUGE part of communications between people in relationships and people looking for relationships. And what's more, is that it AIN'T going away any time soon.

So, it's time to embrace this modern form of communication and use it to our advantage. You need this report because texting can most definitely **MAKE** or **BREAK** your chances with great new guys that you're dating!

Inside you will learn:

- Why texting can BREAK your chances with him
- Why texting can MAKE your chances with him
- What you're probably doing wrong NOW
- The Benefits of texting
- How to make him CRAVE you through texts
- What NOT to send him
- Why you should NEVER sext message or send dirty pictures
- What your PURPOSE should be when texting
- Get ready to gouge his EYES OUT
- Top flirty texts
- Why this isn't a GAME
- The power of implication
- Building tension and why you need to
- Being a NICE bitch
- Silence.
- Texts that really FUCK IT UP
- NEEDYNESS?
- FEAR and texting

I don't want to bore you with too many formalities and bullet points. Let's get straight into this and the first thing we need to take a look at is:

(Please bear in mind that the assumption of this book is that the guy has already shown SOME form of interest in you. After all, you are not going to be texting random men out of the blue, I hope.)

What's the AIM of the texting game?

Not only does that rhyme, but it's the BIG question we need to ask ourselves.

Why do we text each other?

The purpose of texting is simple: to ENGAGE and PROVOKE each other into emotional responses that ultimately help you determine if you're a good match for one another.

And why else? For EXCITEMENT.

It's as simple as that – and it's what life is all about: excitement. If you can find excitement with a man through texting, then you have a sure-fire way of ending up in a great relationship

And believe me, you can GAIN a lot of respect, attention and trust through texting alone. If you aren't playing the texting game well, then you could be shit out of luck.

Let's summarise the aim of the texting game:

-   To engage one another
-   To provoke emotional responses (the right type)
-   To have fun and EXCITEMENT
-   To create sexual tension
-   To LEARN about each other

But if you don't achieve the points above in the correct manner, then you're really gonna screw things up. Which leads us to the next chapter:

Why texting can BREAK your chances with him

Ladies! From the day we are born we become the masters of flirting – and over years and years of practice, we've subconsciously become experts at winning the battle of the sexes (when it comes to flirtation and dating) – BUT...

Whilst text communication has been around for some time, we still haven't come anywhere close to mastering it – and believe it or not – but if you're not doing it right, then you are plain old fuckin' up your chances with men.

Let's take a look at why texting can be the end of your chances with him.

You text him way too much – I know the temptation after you meet a great guy. You want to give your thumbs a good work out and try and figure out as soon as possible when you can see him again.

But doing this can totally screw things up.

You text him the WRONG things – I will cover this entirely throughout the course, so don't panic! But if you are texting your man the wrong things, you can almost certainly mess up ANY chance you have with him through text alone.

It's sad that relationships can be ruined through a text message, but that's just how modern society is!

You don't know when to text him – A tricky ones this – but at what point should YOU be the one to text him? Texting a guy at the WRONG time can be disastrous, make you seem needy and ruin your chances with him.

Again, chill; this will all be sorted later in the book!

You don't know which conversations to have in person, and which in text – The amount of times I've seen women do this is unreal – and it's usually the final nail in the coffin.

Knowing which issues to text your man, and which to leave for phone calls and face-to-face is VITAL for keeping your hopes alive with him.

You're a dirty little girl – Flirting in texts is FINE and part of the fun. And whilst sending naked pictures of yourself or 'sexting' may seem like a good idea, and no doubt he will LOVE it; it's just a TERRIBLE idea and doesn't need to be part of the plan. We will take a look at this section later.

It's just BORING – The whole idea of texting a guy you like is to engage and have fun, right? Well, a lot of girls fuck this up by asking mundane, shitty questions that no man really wants to answer.

Later on we will take a look at some examples of boring texts and some that are exciting.

Why texting can MAKE things happen with him

Okidoke, so we've taken a look at the MANY reasons why texting can mess things up. And I know, there are a lot – but don't panic, they can all be easily avoided and we will cover each point through the course.

Now, let's take a look at why texting can MAKE things between you and your guy even more awesome.

Getting the upper hand – Yep, believe it or not – but you can take complete CONTROL over how things pan out between you and a guy through texting alone.

Using the methods outlined in this course, you should be able to take full control of the man and make him want you like mad.

Creating DESIRE – Again, very easily achieved through text. Creating an even more desirable image of yourself IS NOT achieved through dirty texts and pictures of your privates. There's a TECHIQUE to doing so – and you will learn it soon. Keep reading, you lovely person.

Creating desire = making him want YOU.

Arranging dates – If you know what you're doing, then arranging dates whilst making it seem like his idea is very possible. And if you follow the steps in this book, you should be able to get him to ask you out in no time.

This is POWER, this puts you in control of him, and whilst keeping him happy thinking that he's the one in charge (as men love to be).

But, again – you've got to know the right time to make this happen,

Creating EXCITEMENT – Men love excitement just as much as we do. They CRAVE it and by God they will get bored of you if you aren't giving them it.

Again life is about EXCITEMENT and texting is no exception.

The chase – In none of my books do I ever teach people to play 'mind-games' or anything childish like that. But here, in terms of texting; they need to be the ones chasing us.

Men love a CHALLENGE and texting can create a huge mental challenge for men that they will try and win. Getting a guy to be the one who chases you and seeks your attention is vital for pushing things to the next level with him.

As I say, games are a big NO NO in my book, but there are a few subtle methods we can utilize to make sure we are the ones he thinks about when he gets into his bed at night.

All that being said – let's get into the meat of the book, and start with our first issue:

When should I text him?

Let's start from square one.

You've met a guy, hung out, had a date, whatever.

You like him, and he's showed an interest in you by giving you his number. Great!

But now, what next? As we discussed above, the temptation is to text him as soon as you get home or even the next day. In an ideal world, he will text you first – but you need to give him the chance to text you first. You want to be the one being chased, not the other way around!

If he DOES NOT text you after a week or meeting, then it's time to start thinking about making the first move. In most cases, you will only need to wait 3 days before he texts you first.

When a man gets home after a date, he EXPECTS the girl to text him pretty promptly – and in most cases this does happen. But what does this do? Well, it does nothing for your chances with him, and here's why.

Most men will go through a tonne of dates before finding the right girl to commit to. And that's because there is no challenge for them. Men love a challenge; they NEED to EARN something in order to respect it – and relationships with women are no exception.

So while all his other girls are texting him up after dates with him, you can be sat there quietly, getting into his head.

'Why hasn't she text me yet?'

'Didn't I impress her enough?'

'I'd better find out what she's up to'

The three things that will go through a guys mind if you play it cool and DON'T text him. This will work in most cases – it's just how men are.

You've now become a challenge to him, which means he's going to start showing more interest in you.

What if he doesn't text me after a week?

Well, in that case he needs a little more from you. He may NOT have been blown away by your initial date/first meet. Believe it or not...

BUT – that's fine. There's only so much you can learn about a person after meeting them once. There is still plenty of time to gain his attention and attraction.

There is of course the possibility that he is trying to play the waiting game as well – but in general, 3 days will feel like an eternity for him.

In most cases, if he interested even the slightest, he will hit you up in good time.

Here's what needs to happen if he doesn't

First off – don't directly ask him out on a date. It's needy – and we will discuss being needy later. For now, just know not to do it.

Example ALERT

You: *'Hi. Want to go out again on Saturday with me?'*

Him: *'Sure- why not.'*

Seems good enough, right? Wrong! While you may have scored yourself a date with the guy, it was by no means easy for him to obtain. And remember: men do NOT value things that they haven't earned – and you are GIVING him yourself with this type of text.

Plus, it's just plain fucking **BORING.** You want to create **EMOTION**, not boredom.

Let's take a look at an example that you should consider using:

You: *'Crazy night the other night at Danny's- you light weight! :P – can't believe what my friends said about you!'*

Him: *'It was mad! Me? lightweight? What did they say?!'*

This is a GREAT start! You've provoked an emotional response, started an interesting conversation and filled him with CURIOUSTY. But where do you go from here?

You: *'Oh nothing much ;) – we are all heading out Saturday at 9 if you wanna find out! Not sure if I've got a lift there yet though'*

Him: *'Sure, I'll be there! I can pick you up at 8!'*

Ok – this is good. Now let's bullet point why this is good and summarise what you need to have achieved with your initial texts.

- Some form of **CHALLENGE/HUMOUR** – *'you light weight!'*
- Curiosity – *'Can't believe what my friends said about you!'*
- Relatable reference – *'at Danny's'*
- Mystery – *'Oh nothing much ;)'*
- Be friendly/light

CREATE: **CHALLENGE**, **CURIOUSITY**, **REFERANCE** and **MYSTERY**

Next comes the actual process in which you get him to take you out on a date. You aren't asking him to come out with you – you are giving him the OPTION to join you if he wants – but of course he wants to after all the emotions we've created already.

- Give him the OPTION to join you, never ask.
- Give him the time and day
- Add a little more intrigue as incentive to get him out *'if you wanna find out!'*
- The more humour you can add, the better – but don't force it.
- Give him a reason to come and pick YOU up - like it's HIS idea. The *'I've not got a lift'* line works a treat.

So, while that seems long-winded; ALWAYS try and include the above aspects into your texts if you are the one texting him first. The point is to prod his ego, provoke his emotions, challenge him and make him laugh.

The more emotion you create, the better.

ALWAYS TRY TO:

CREATE EXCITEMENT

MAKE REFERENCE

USE HUMOUR

&

CHALLENGE

What to do if he DOES text FIRST

Now, this being the most likely of the two events – but still needs to handled with properly in order to create the same emotions as we did above. Let's take a look at an example of the wrong type of text to send.

Him: *'Hi sexy, had a nice time on Friday. Want to come out again on Saturday?'*

You: *'Yes!!! When and where?'*

Him: *'Rockers at 9, pick you up at 8!'*

You: *'Ok perfect, can't wait!'*

Meeeeh – whilst you have got the first text you wanted and a date with him, it doesn't say much about you. It says you're the type of person who will jump at the chance to see him and most likely drop anything to go out with him.

Whilst it may create a bit of excitement for him knowing that you will take him up on pretty much any offer (probably thinking he will get sex too), it just doesn't create the challenge and emotion that we REALLY want to gain respect.

R.E.S.P.E.C.T

As well as creating emotion and challenge, we need to earn RESPECT. And he needs to respect that he can't just have you whenever he wants. And the more respect you earn, the more desirable person you will become.

Here's a better example:

Him: *'Hi sexy, had a nice time on Friday. Want to come out again on Saturday?'*

You: *Hey cutie! That does sound amazing, but I'm a little tied up this whole weekend. I'm free Wednesday at 7 if you like??'*

Him: *'Sure! That's great I will text you closer to that time to arrange pick up'*

Ok, this is pretty good. Whilst it doesn't create too much emotion, it does however leave the impression that you are a BUSY person who priorities her own life above men. And that is an INSTANT respect gainer.

But at the same time you structure your text to make yourself sound generally interested in him:

- You seem excited to get a text from him

- You compliment him 'cutie'
- You arrange a solid date and time that you are free
- And now guaranteed more texts from him in between meeting, which allows time to create more emotion and excitement for the night.

Now, there are ways to provoke some emotional feelings here too, but that depends how risky you want to be with your texts. Here's another example that will get your man thinking and dying to see you.

Him: *'Hi sexy, had a nice time on Friday. Want to come out again on Saturday?'*

You: *'Hey beautiful! That sounds awesome! But my friend is staying over the whole weekend. How about 7pm on Tuesday instead? Are you sure you can handle those tequilas??'*

Him: *'Oh! Ok yeh cool – see you then!'*

This – this is my favourite type of text to send a guy. But it needs to be worded very carefully as it contains a lot of emotional triggers that will make his head fuzz.

So what's so effective about this type of text?

- Again, you come across as being BUSY
- You have a 'friend' staying over. His first thoughts will be that it's another guy you are seeing, which will create some **emotion**, curiosity and a little jealously if his mind takes him that far.
- You set the date that YOU want, not him.
- And you set a challenge with a little humour *'Are you sure you can handle those tequilas??'*

Let's get one thing straight: I HATE playing mind games, and I never resort to them. Telling a guy that you're with a friend is borderline with that though – but it creates the curiosity and busy feeling that we are looking for. Also, a little bit of jealousy is natural – if he can't handle even that then he's not a keeper.

You just have to make sure you don't cross that line when it comes to jealousy. It's truly a terrible thing and can wreak havoc on some people's mind. **For example:**

Him: *'Come out with me on Saturday?'*

You: *'No can do buddy! Staying with my hot friend Tom for the weekend. Maybe another time, eh?'*

Way WAY too much negative emotions attached to this type of message. And frankly if you're the type of person to try and provoke a male this far, then you're a bitch, frankly.

Men can get just as insecure as us women, and prodding at his fragile ego like this is going to put him well off you. If he thinks you're the type of girl that going to make him feel insecure and not good about himself, then he won't come running to you ever again.

The goal is to BUILD bonds between the two of you, not break them before things have even started.

This leads me to my next smallish chapter:

THINK BEFORE YOU TEXT

Doesn't rhyme, but still needs to be discussed.

That's the HUGE advantage texting has over talking to someone in person or on the phone: you have time to THINK. There is no pressure to come up with an answer straight away – and by God USE this to your advantage.

It's so easy to fuck your chances up by not thinking and sending the wrong type of text. We women are very emotional and are actions are based on these emotions, not through correct thinking.

Let's take for example if you were the one asking him out first (through the methods in the book)

Example:

You: *'Crazy night the other night at Danny's- you light weight! :P – can't believe what my friends said about you!'*

Him: *'It was mad! Me? Lightweight? What did they say?!'*

You: *'Oh nothing much ;) – we are all heading out Saturday at 9 if you wanna find out! Not sure if I've got a lift there yet though'*

Him: *'Hmm, I can't think week because my friend Jess is down for a couple days. Next week is cool though!'*

EMOTIONAL REPLY:

You: *'Right OK – who is this Jess person then?! You should come out with me still'*

Him: *NO REPLY*

 Terrible reply, and sadly loads of women text from emotion like this. It's needy and needy is very unattractive. Let's take a look at how you should reply to texts like this.

THINKERS REPLY:

You: *'Ok cool! No prob – give me a shout next week if you get free. Have fun!'*

Him: *'Will do! I'll drop you a text later or something!'*

You: DON'T REPLY

This is more like it. You're letting him do his own this, with his own people – and you're not making anything of it. You're playing the whole 'cool, I don't care what you do' card. Even if you have your suspicion that he's up to naughty things, just be cool and wish him a good time!

Then leave his reply alone. He will be expecting you to reply, but he knows now that he can see you next week, and he will damn sure go through with it.

Ok, speaking of needy – that brings me to the next section of the book – AFTER I SHARE WITH YOU SOME SECRET TEXTS!

Top 8 AFTER DATE TEXTS

Ladies get ready to create all the emotion, tension, excitement and intrigue you need to hook your man. Here are my favourite 8 texts to send after a date with a man.

'That was a HOT night at Jennie's right? Shame you couldn't get me much hotter...'

'I don't think I've ever seen a guy pull off the 'Drunken Monkey' look before – well done! ☺'

'So funny what my friends had to say about you! ;) Can't believe they said you were sexy :P..'

'Looked like most girls there had their eye on you that night! Shame, I found it quite easy to take them off you! ☺'

'You looked cute last night – shame about what my friends told me though! ;) '

'What was the cologne you wore last night? Kinda reminded me of dog shit! Shame, cuz you definitely didn't look like dog shit...;)'

'Take no notice of what they been saying about you! I thought you looked dead sexy!!'

'It's funny how no one liked that 'dance' of yours the other night. Maybe you can teach me a few moves?! :D'

MAKE SURE YOU VARY YOUR TEXTS!!

There is a risky level of humour involved in some of these texts. If your guy can't see that you're joking and takes huge offence by a joke text, LOOK OUT. You, and only you can weigh up whether your guy can take a joke or not – so just be careful.

Being needy in your texts

Being needy is one of the number one 'chance killers' when it comes to texting. Yes, you can say whatever you want through a text message without having the hassle of facing someone in person. But trust me; being needy is a total turn off - a MASSIVE turn off.

Do you know what men find really attractive in women?

- Women who are independent
- Women who have goals in life
- Women with self respect
- Women with humour
- Women WITHOUT emotional baggage

Read this next example of a text and then I will ask you a question about it.

Him: *'Yeh that's cool, we can hang out again soon'*

You: *'Ok, when???'*

Him: *'Not sure yet, kinda busy'*

You: *'Well, I wanna do it again soon'*

Him: *'Ok, I will let you know when I get free!'*

You: *'Can't you find out sooner? Like tomorrow?'*

Him: NOOOO REPLY....

Now let me ask you: does the above make 'You' sound like an independent, respectable, baggage-free, fun-loving and humorous person?

NO – OBVIOUSLY NOT.

I know, I know – the temptation is ALWAYS there to try and push things and make them happen as soon as you can. But sticking to the texting guidelines in this course will give you the upper hand; I can assure you of that.

Neediness pushes men away, and if you act needy, you will push that guy away. Neediness then becomes desperation, which of course leads to double texting.

Double-texting

So you were needy and didn't get the reply you wanted – well done, not! The worst thing you can do now is follow up with a double-text which then makes you look even needier. Imagine the text conversation above followed by:

You: '*Why didn't you text me back?*'

Him: '*Was busy...*'

Ok, if a guy wants to text you back - he WILL. And even if he comes back with an 'I was busy' type of reply – it's usually bullshit to try and stop you texting even more.

Being needy isn't creating any sort of positive desire or emotion. However, you are challenging him; challenging his patience with you. He probably won't put up with much, especially after you've just met. He's going to think you are emotionally unstable and ditch your ass!

The thought of spending time with a needy person is a real turn off.

- Stay cool
- Think before you text
- Do everything in your power to not seem needy
- Any emotional issues you have need to be resolved before you start dating

And that's true. If you have got some **emotional problems**, especially after a hard breakup, then you need to sort them out first. Hiding these types of emotions is going to be hard and will cloud your judgement, causing irrational texts that screw things up and make you feel even shitter.

What can stop me feeling needy?

I get asked this question a lot – and it's got everything to do with your current lifestyle. Sometimes the temptation to be what is considered 'needy' is overwhelming and nearly uncontrollable.

But the good news is that it is controllable, and you need to fix this before jumping into anything with a man.

Being needy is about relying on other people to make you feel wanted. You want your guy to drop everything and go out with you, because it will make you feel like a worthy person, right?

BUT, the focus here has nothing to do with him; it's all about you. The only thing you should NEED is to need your life to improve and be where you want to be. TRUE happiness won't come from having a guy want to be with you.

True happiness will come from pursuing the dreams in your life and striving to be the best YOU can be – and when you focus on achieving that, only then will you NOT feel the need to get needy with men. Men will WANT you, and they will want you BAD.

Once you set your mind on the REAL priorities in life, you won't feel like you need to gain acceptance from a man.

- Join a gym
- Pursue a hobby
- Pursue a career

Ask yourself: where do I want to be in a year's time? Focus on that and the relations with men will flow naturally and become even more enjoyable.

Ok, this isn't a course on bettering your life, but it was important for stopping them God awful needy texts. So, let's get back on track and take a look at something a little SPICIER.

Flirtation in texts

Flirting is FUN!

And flirting in text messages can create a lot of desire and positive emotions from your man, if you know how to do it!

You need to bear in mind that there is a difference between flirting and sending dirty text messages or pictures of yourself.

Flirting can create a beautiful sexual tension, create excitement and intrigue WHILST keeping your respect intact. And that's VITAL for future relations with men; you need to keep your respect intact at all times!

Whilst it may seem like a saucy little surprise to send a guy a dirty text message or a nude picture of you, it just isn't a good idea.

While it's certainly and OK thing to do when in a full-blown relationship, you don't want to do it right off the bat. The message you are giving out is that you are an easy slut who he is able to bed whenever he wants. Want kind of woman would want to give out that type of message? Also, the main thing you are losing here is respect for yourself – and once you text him something dirty, there will be no end to it back from him.

This removes any limitations he may feel between the two of you. Men will JUMP at the chance to get into bed with you, and this is the exact signal you are sending off with those types of messages.

With that being said, let's take a look at a few examples that will create **DESIRE** and positive **EMOTION** from your guy.

STOP! Example time.

Him: 'You look really sexy in that dress last night btw...'

You: 'Thanks, I think it would suit you better! Although that t-shirt really made your arms look really sexy. I can picture them around me... ;) – you probably don't hit the gym too often though...:P'

This is good, and let's takes a look why it's good and what needs to be achieved in flirty messages.

-   You took the compliment with a simple 'Thanks'
-   Didn't resort to anything too sexual, keeping limitation in place
-   And respect still intact
-   You complimented him, and triggered an arousing emotion by calling his arms sexy.
-   And then you added the challenge at the end, suggesting he looked good but doubted his ability in the gym.

When you get a compliment, TAKE IT. Don't go fishing for more compliments or ask why you looked sexy or whatever. This makes it sound like you don't already know that you are attractive, which makes you seem like you lack the confidence to believe it. And remember: confidence is sexy!

Never overstep the flirtation. NEVER. Well, until you are in a committed relationship – but if you give off the impression you get 'dirty' after the first date, then he's going to lose respect for you and wonder how many other men you talk to like that...

You can drive a man WILD through these suggestive texts alone. Even more so than sending full-on dirty messages. His mind will run wild at the thoughts you plant in there.

As for the 'challenge' – you've got to be very careful with this. Whilst it can come across humorous and trigger a response from him, it can also come across badly. And that's the next section I want to talk about.

Text misinterpretation

Yep, texting is one hell of an easy way to come across as an absolute jerk, even if you didn't mean it. And once that happens it's hard to come back from.

In this section we will take a look at a very special ways to make sure your little jokes don't come across as being hurtful or offensive.

Remember: people read texts AS IF they were being SAID by you, and even the slightest of errors can make you sound like a dick.

How to avoid potential offence

Him: '*Yen well yak know, I've been hitting the gym lately*'

You: '*Really, it doesn't show*'

While you may just be joking around, suggesting he obviously does go enough; this can easily sound bitchy and rude. Here's how to reply to such a text the right way.

Him: '*Yeh well ya know, I've been hitting the gym lately*'

You: '*Oh really?! It doesn't show! ;)*'

That's more like it. Most men will be able to take it for the blatant joke it is, especially after you've just complimented him on his physique.

If you find that your guy can't take jokes like this, or misinterprets everything you say to him as an insult, then maybe he's too insure for you.

All it takes is a cheeky face, or emoticon as they are know, and an exclamation mark to make it read the way you want it to sound.

You've got emoticons; feel free to use them to your advantage to show a man how he should be interpreting your texts! ☺

Read your text first before sending them. **THINK**. Does it read the way it needs to sound? Don't fuck up your chances with him by sending something that can be easily misinterpreted! ☹

Even the simplest of altercations to your text can come across differently in a man's mind. Take this for example:

You: Hey – how was last night with your buddies?'

Him: 'Yeh good thanks'

That's cool that you're showing an interested in him and his friends, but does it sound sincere? How about...

You: Hey! Did you have fun with ya buddies last night!? ☺'

Him: INSERT REPLY HERE

That's much more engaging! That exclamation mark at the end of 'Hey' really makes it sound like you're interested in saying hi to him. And the exclamation mark and question mark at the end create a sense of urgency that make it seem like you REALLY care about his evening with buddies.

And to top it off, the smiley face makes it seem even more legitimate.

You get the point, right? You need to take the time when you craft a text message to make sure it comes across as legitimate and exciting as possible, even if it's a simple little text. He is taking note of everything you send him! It makes you that little bit more friendly and easier to engage with- trust me!

Always be careful, but remember to always be...

CONFIDENTLY DOES IT

Confidence is SEXY as hell – and men love it. In fact, I can bet right now that you love a confident man, right? It goes both ways. And it's vital that you come across as confident in your text messages too.

Confidence makes you seem in control of your life, and maybe in slightly daring in the things you can get away with saying – and in text messages, it's vital.

Imagine your typical 'bitch'. Men love these bitches because they act confident, seem self-reliant and generally in control of all situations. Think of yourself to become a kind of...mini, tongue in cheek bitch.

You want to have the confident aspects, but you don't want to come across as rude, pushy or arrogant like bitches do.

The type of humour you use in your texts can really determine how confident you come across. I tend to use a 'daring' type of humour to assert my confidence in ways that most can't, through texting. Here are some examples of what I mean:

Him: '*You smelt amazing last night! What was the perfume?*'

You: '*It was Calvin Klein. What was yours? Eu De Dog Shit!?* ☺'

This is daring, and if done correctly, can come across as confident. It shows confidence in being able to say something crude but with humour – something most people are not confident enough to do.

More importantly, it again, forces an emotional reaction from him, challenges his and contains a humorous element.

This needs to be performed correctly or can come across as rude through text. For example:

Him: '*You smelt amazing last night! What was the perfume?*'

You: '*Well you smelt like dog shit.*'

Remember how easily texts can sound if worded wrong? Take note of the use of humour to emphasise the overall joke; the smiley emoticon used and the correct use of punctuation.

And again, THINK before you send this type of text. If you weren't joking around with him like this on your first date, and it appears he can handle a joke in person, then you should probably avoid sending texts like this to him.

If you word it correctly, your confidence will SHINE through, making you that little bit more attractive.

DON'T be nervous when you text. He is probably nervous to text you things like that too – but once you break down this barrier, you will both have a much more exciting and free-flowing time when texting each other.

But of course, you need to know WHEN to make jokes and which conversations need to be had in person, not through text.

When you should talk face-to-face

Texting is easy – and it's very tempting to talk about serious issues that you are too shy to converse about in person. But, it's not a good idea – ever. Texting about issues between the two of you can create an uncomfortable tension when in person. And since most issues will be that of a negative nature, things can get misinterpreted very easily, which can lead to all kinds of problems.

Such matters as:

- 'Are we a couple yet?' Doesn't need to be asked in a text – and in fact, this should come naturally.
- 'I wish you'd feel the same way about me as I do you' – again, avoid taking this route through text. If you have a serious emotional question that you need answering, talk about it in person.
- 'I don't want to see you anymore' – Ok, most people will do this through text – but please, have some respect for your SO or the person you are dating, and do this in person.
- 'Do you love me?' – Such a weird text to receive. And definitely one that needs to be shared in person, face-to-face. And ideally, he will be the one saying it to you first!
- 'I'm worried about...your health/job/family/etc' – anything that you are worried about regarding your man needs to be discussed in person. Chances are that he may not want to talk about them anyway.
- ARUGEMENTS – make sure you never get into a lengthy argument in a text message. Not only does it make you sound like a teenager, but it also makes it a lot easier to say very hurtful things...If you find yourself getting toward that way, either stop texting or defuse the situation with humour.

Example:

Him: 'You looked totally sexy last night!

You: 'Wish I could say the same about you. You kinda looked like a mole in a suit!'

Him: 'What!?'

WRONG

You: *'Don't worry'*

You: *'Sorry didn't mean that in a bad way'*

RIGHT

You: *'I mean like, an INCREDIBLY SEXY mole in a suit...;) haha!'*

This could have easily escalated through a dented ego – just make sure you are quick to defuse the situation before anything further comes of it.

Which reminds me: **STOP** saying 'sorry'.

You know, saying 'sorry' too much makes you look weak. You don't need to apologise for every single text that someone misinterprets. You knew that you weren't trying to be offensive so there is no need to say sorry. If you feel there is a point where you need to say sorry, then just try and defuse the issue again with humour.

You never know through text. He might not have been offended at all by what you said - so instantly apologising is going to kill any fun that conversation could have led to. If you have TRUELY offended him out of spite, then you will need to apologise.

And then again, in person.

Hey – wanna know how to kill off your chances with him without being mean, rude, bitchy, possessive or overly nice?

LIKE DIS

Ok so lyk dis chapter am gna shw u how u cn relli fuk fings up between u n a new fella. Its pretti simpl relli – all u gtta do is strt txting like dis...

Ok, I can't bring myself to write like that any further without clawing my eyes out of my skull – but I will assume you get the point.

I will also assume that if you are reading this that you are aged 18 or age. And in that case, you should by now have gone passed that horrible phase of 'text chat' that I so poorly demonstrated above.

Why shouldn't you text like this? Well, it makes you seem like a teenager still. That's how children and immature women talk – and no self-respecting, desirable man is going to be interesting in holding a text conversation with you if you text like that.

In fact, I think it's nearly impossible to text like this now, given the amount of auto-correction keypads that are used on phones these days! If you can use them, then do it. Structure your sentences like an intelligent female, not a squeaky voiced teenager.

Do ya undastand?

Plus, it's really fucking annoying...

Rememba:

not 2 make ya

TXTS lk like dis or

ur man gna leev you

4 sum1 whoo aint

sounding lyk a

MORON

Earning respect

Respect is something that is **EARNT.**

If a man thinks he is able to walk all over you and get what he wants from you, when he wants, he will most likely try to.

To earn respect, you have to stop these things from being able to take place at the word GO, right from the start – and it's actually pretty easy to do.

The first way a woman loses her respect is by sleeping with a man after a first date or meeting. The man will think he can get 'some of that' whenever he wants, and will most likely try to. This leads to a purely sexual relationship developing and not an emotional one.

You have to make it obvious from day ONE that you are NOT that girl. And if he can't handle not getting his way with you, then he's a possessive, controlling asshole. Simple. If he starts texting you excessively dirty messages, then you need to defuse them as soon as you can without sounding uptight.

Example:

Him: '*Wow you looked hot last night. Would really love to fuck you..How about it?.'*

You: '*Oh wow, prince charming I see! ;) I'm sure it would be good, but that's something you need to earn ☺'*

There is nothing wrong with letting him know he has to earn your body before he can have it. But notice you were not dismissive or harsh in your message, and even added a little humour, whilst suggesting it probably would be good.

If he continues to proposition you with sex and is what is known as a 'sex pest' then he may not be ready for a relationship. Let's not hate on the entire male race for this. Most guys are like this and it's in their nature. Some however, will be prepared to earn it from you whilst respecting the boundaries you have set.

And as we discussed earlier, gaining respect comes from creating a reasonable boundary between the two of you. Achieved by:

- Not giving him sex when HE wants it
- Putting your life before his

- Making him earn you
- Having goals in life that aren't about him
- Being confident
- Not being needy

And that is the basics to EARNING RESPECT. It's not hard and really doesn't take much practice.

Once a man see's that you are a respectable person, he will start to treat you like one. Which will usually lead to more sexual tension, more exciting conversations, and hopefully many more dates.

And remember, respect is something that a man will love to show off. The thought of having a classy, confident and respectful looking female on his arm is very appealing. A great way to separate yourself from the riff-raff!

Aaaaaaand that's all for this section ladies – time to press on with the next side of things!

What Turns Men OFF

Hello there – it's me again, Melanie Raymund!

Welcome to my next report 'What turns men off' – and inside this report, ladies, we will be taking a look at two CRUCIAL issues:

- What turns men **OFF** in general
- What turns men **OFF** in bed

And THAT'S IT.

For centuries now, women just like you and me have pondered over the reasoning behind men suddenly and seemingly unreasonably becoming turned off.

Do not FEAR.

Times have changed and men are easier to read than ever. And in this report, we will take an EXACT look at what turns men off in and out of bed, and how you can AVOID becoming that turn off.

Read this REPORT if you want to make sure you AVOID all possible TURN OFFS

Ok, sit back, break out the chocolates and enjoy my very special report!

Let's get started.

What turns men off in general?

Despite the vast majority of the female population believing that men are just damn dirty apes who will fuck anything that walks, they are actually human as well and get turned off just as fast as we do in NON bed-related situations.

Have you ever started dated a guy and things were going swimmingly and then suddenly...

Nothing.

No texting, no calls – no contact whatsoever.

What went wrong? You didn't even do that weird vaginal fart thing in bed (more on that later) – so why the sudden change of heart?

Well, believe it or not, there are a number of non sexual reasons that can turn your man off faster than the above! Let's break the top reasons down and analyse how you can avoid such mistakes in the future and keep your man ON.

Turn off number one – Neediness

I've made 3 awesome Kindle books now (you may own the others) and in each of them I have a section about neediness, and how terribly unattractive it really is. And the reason I talk about it so much, is because it really is THAT BAD.

No matter if you are in a relationship or just dating, neediness is a huge turn off for a guy. While some girls might like the thought of a guy being there every waking second that she needs him; guys don't operate on the same level.

'I need to see you tonight'

'Let's do something this weekend. When are you free? I want to see you'

'I'm upset and lonely, cheer me up'

Unless your man is dying to get his end away, persistent neediness is going to kill his hardon faster than he can say his own name.

Here's what you are doing right now that turns him off:

- Constant texting
- Constant calling
- Constantly needing to meet up

- Not giving him his own time
- Craving his attention more than other things in your life
- Freaky Facebook posts

Regardless of whether you are in a relationship with him or just dating, you need to just 'BE COOL' – and take the time to focus on your own life, not his.

Remember: Want him, but don't NEED him.

How to avoid this turn off: Simple. Don't be needy.

Turn off number two – Sharing too much

You know those 'girly' conversations that you have with your female buddies? The ones were you openly talk about every gritty issue of your daily life?

Keep them between you and your girls.

Men don't want hear about your problems, especially ones that come from your own body. What we've become used to talking about over the years is like nails on a chalk board to men. They don't know about it, and they don't want to know about it.

Like these:

- Anything regarding your period
- Unexplainable emotional issues
- How much you hate 'that' girl
- Other men.

Other men? A man's ego is as fragile as our own, and can be easily broken at the thought of a superior man in your life. No man wants to know about that 'hot' guy you were dating before, or the one that you got in to bed last week.

Here's some solid advice. DON'T talk about your ex's. It brings the conversation to an 'it's all about me' feeling and really isn't interesting to talk about. Never compare your ex to your new fella.

And NEVER try to use one guy to make another one jealous. It may work well in the short-run, but soon he will get fed up and the turn off will be so immense that he will ditch your ass and move on.

Oh by the way: it's generally OK to talk about that crush you have on 'that' celebrity. If he can't handle that, then he has some major self-esteem issues.

How to avoid this turn off: THINK before you start a conversation about one of 'those' things. Men don't want to talk about your bloody vagina and another other process taking part in your body that he can't wrap his mind around.

Find yourself a MALE friend and ask him which things he hates talking about with his girlfriend. You will be surprised how much you can learn from a guy.

Turn off number three – 5 Year Plan?

This is totally scary for a lot of guys, especially if you have only just started dating – and I'm hoping big time that you aren't one of these people.

Planning out a future between you and your new man is a huge turn off, and one big enough to send him packing. Men LOVE their freedom and the thought of having their future planned for them is damn scary.

Whilst men are definitely willing to commit to long-term relations, there is something very smothering about the thought of losing the things he loves doing:

- Spending time with friends
- Going out drinking
- Playing sports

Whilst of course these things are still maintainable whilst in a relationship, coming on so strong with a 'plan' for the two of you so early can make it seem like you will be eliminating the fun from his life.

How to avoid this turn off: Take things slowly when you first start dating him. Don't give him any indication that there is any sort of 'plan' for things between you, even if you have one in your mind!

Turn off number four – Talking too much

Yak yak yak.

Us girls, we LOVE to yak, spread rumours and just generally gossip. And that's where you may just be turning him off.

Have you ever been around a group of men and noticed the way they talk? The pace is much slower and relaxed. The temptation you may have, is to start talking to him as if he were one of your girlfriends.

DON'T.

Keep the pace somewhere between slow and medium, as much as it may pain you to do so. Men enjoy conversation the most when it's not so 'back-and-forth' at a crazy pace.

- Slow down
- Don't just talk about yourself
- Be humorous more than serious
- Engage with him on his level, not yours

I know you would really love to have a good old bitch about that slut at work that you don't get on with – but your man doesn't want to hear about it, even if he shows some interest, it's not a turn on for him whatsoever.

Try talking about things that BOTH of you like, that way the pace of the conversation will become more neutral to both your likings.

How to avoid this turn off: Hold yourself back from talking about every damn issue in your life. Emotional issues are the biggest drag of them all, but are very easy to rant on and on about.

Keep the pace low and you won't scare him off.

Turn off number five – FUCK, SHIT.

Whilst you may be using naughty words to emphasise your point, swearing too much is a turn off for men. Sure, you've heard men talking to each other and they seems to be a 'fuck' or 'shit' used every other word – but we are ladies.

Men want to be associated romantically with ladies, and female attributes, not male ones. And constant swearing is definitely a male attribute.

'Yeh that bad last night was fucking awesome! We should go see them again'

'Holy fucking fuck! That bad was THE shit last night. Who the fuck thought they could be so shitting awesome?'

Yes, it's time to use a swear word to emphasise your point every now and then, but take a look how stupid and 'buddy-like' you would sound if you swore too much.

How to avoid this turn off: Moderate your swearing. Even if you think it makes you sound like a bad-ass female gangster, just DON'T do it. The less you swear the better. And trust me, this DOES turn men OFF.

Turn off number six – Smoking

Personally, I don't smoke. At all.

But if you do, that's fine – but please realise that having that 'smoky' smell around your body is a massive turn off, for SOME men. Notice how I didn't say ALL men. I've been around some men who actually enjoy the smell of a smoky lady – but trust me; these are the type of men you want to be attracting.

Like most smokers, you don't realise it – but after you have a smoke, you STINK – and even if you think you've got the smell off your clothes, it's still there on your breath.

Picture yourself waiting at home in your sexy lingerie; the imminent arrival of your wonder man and the excitement of that first kiss you will share when he arrives.

You're patiently waiting and decide to have a quick smoke to ease the nerves. Ok it's finished and you freshen up a little bit as half an hour goes by. He arrives!

You kiss passionately as he enters your humble abode.

Then, out of the blue, he throws up on you, panics, rushes out the front door and drives home never to be seen again.

Ok, admittedly that is likely to never happen – but trust me, that smell of smoke is STILL on your breath and kissing someone with smoky breath is quite disgusting. Even if you can't 'smell' your own breath, trust me, IT IS STILL THERE and it WILL turn him off.

How to avoid this turn off: A no-brainer here: don't smoke! Of course, easier said than done. But you definitely give yourself at least one hour of 'recovery' time after having a smoke. If you have tooth paste and mouthwash at your disposal, then make sure to God that you use it before you start getting intimate.

Turn off number seven – Acne

Again, this is something a man will most likely never admit to – but having bad skin is a turn off for guys! It's very sad that our society now deems something as uncontrollable as skin conditions a turn-off, but that's just the way it is.

When a man looks at you, he looks at how soft your skin is. Why? Because it's normal for men to think about being pressed up very close to you in a sexual way, even if you are meeting for the first time (classic men). And of course, when he's up close to you, he isn't going to want to be staring back at a face full of puss.

There are a few ways you can 'conceal' your imperfections, as I'm sure you and your make-up kit are aware. But the real beauty behind your skin comes naturally and that type of attractiveness isn't something that can be achieved through makeup.

I struggled with acne from the ages of 18-24 and it literally ruined my love life due to lack of self-esteem and people not being attracted to a pizza face. There were only a very few methods that actually make my skin clear – and since it's your lucky day, I'm going to share them with you.

Egg white – If you are suffering from acne, then get on the EGG WHITE. Believe me; this is far more effective and cheaper than over the counter products.

All you need to do is separate the white from the yolk and then give the white a good whisking until it's all frothy-like.

Take a paper towel and dip it in the egg white.

Spread it across your face and leave it on for about 15 minutes – 30 at the max.

Rinse off with Luke-warm water and you are done! Do this every day if your skin is very bad, or 3-4 times a week if it's just 'bad'.

Change the pillow case – Not changing your pillow case to a fresh clean one EVERY day is costing your skin.

You see, nasty bacteria build up on your pillow case, and when you sleep, you are pressing your face right in that SHIT, which ultimately causes acne to form or get worse.

Very simple solution: change your pillow case every single night and I promise you will start to notice a change in your skin.

Make-up – As we know, makeup is vital for those of us who want to 'fit in', unfortunately. But you need to make sure that you TAKE IT OFF, when you go to bed. Your skin needs to breathe and when it's suffocated by 3 layers of makeup, it can't! And when it can't breathe, this is where your acne is allowed to fester and become worse.

Take it off before you go to bed and don't wear it unless you absolutely need to!

Nasty products – When you get acne, there is always the temptation to go out and buy chemical-based products. And while SOME have SOME positive effects on SOME people, most of them are shit and will leave your skin worse.

If you need to buy something for your skin, make sure there is NO alcohol in that product as it will dry your skin and make your acne even worse.

I haven't washed my face with soap or a product for YEARS now, and I have totally clear skin. My advice would be to wash with just water or a very gentle skin cleanser. If you do use a cleanser, only use a small amount once a day.

And those are my best tips for acne. Feel free to try them and you will improve your skin condition!

Turn off number 8 – Emotional baggage

Emotional baggage.

You take that shit with you wherever you go, no matter how hard you try and conceal it; it always finds a way to shine through and fuck things up.

There are a BOAT (I actually wrote 'Borat' there first, hehe) load of emotional issues that can turn men off you in a heartbeat. And sharing these issues with him is never a good idea, unless you really feel its holding things back between the two of you. Here are some of them:

- Heartbroken from a previous relationship. While you may still hurt for another guy, this is definitely some serious turn off material for any new guy you may get involved with.
- Family issues.
- Health issues.
- Low self-esteem. There is no bigger turn off than a gal who keeps putting herself down time and time again...

While of course you CAN hide these issues when it comes to dating other men, and hope to God they don't come pouring out; it's not the best solution – because most of the time, they will.

What I would suggest, is that you get yourself into the right frame of mind before you even start considering dating men. Even if this takes you a fair while, it will be worth it. If you run head first into the dating scene and your mind is chock-a-block with emotional drama, you're destined to fail.

And trying to use your new man as an outlet for un-bottling these dramas is sure as hell going to TURN HIM OFF and have him running a mile.

Turn off number nine – Your EX

Ok, I'm going to put this very bluntly in the next sentence.

Men do NOT give a flying FUCK about your stupid-ass ex-boyfriend.

Seriously, they don't want to hear a damn peep about him. There is nothing interesting you can say about your ex that he's going to be interested in or turned on by.

And for the love of God, if you are going to make comparisons between your new guy and your old guy, make sure you are praising the new one. I've actually heard of women telling guys how their EX's used to act and how they should try to be similar to that – unreal.

Let's break this down into some quick bullet points. I'm really hoping most of these are obvious but you'd be amazed by how many women do these things...

- Bragging how much your ex was earning or how exciting his job is.
- Trying to compare penis size. 'Yeh he was the size of a donkey'
- Explaining how physically in shape he was
- How good he was in bed, or things he did to you that you liked 'My ex used to bend me over the kitchen sink, can you?'
- Never ever EVER any mention during sex
- Anything, really – unless you're explaining what a dick he was. And even then, men don't want to hear that too much.

Mentioning his name in a bad light too frequently is just as bad. It makes guys think that you still have some form of emotional connection with him – which if you are always talking about him, then you probably do.

Sort that shit out.

BREAK DOWN

Ok these are generally the top five turn offs for men when it comes to NON sexual turn offs. Let's quick recap on these so you don't forget:

- Neediness
- Sharing too much
- Planning out a future
- Talking too much
- Smokey breath
- Acne
- Swearing

Now it's time to get into the juicy part of the book.

The SEXUAL turn offs!

Brace yourself ladies, it's time to get a little dirty...

What turns men off sexually?

I really don't think that this needs an introduction as both men and women both get turned off from certain things in the sack. However, there are a few differences that may not be so obvious that you NEED to know about.

Ok, so let's drive straight on in a talk about the top turn offs in bed, and how to prevent them!

Turn off number one – It's too sensitive, OUCH!

Yes it's hard to know the exact science and every sensation behind the opposite gender's genitals – but there is one thing that men HATE and will have them turned off from having sex with you for some time. In fact, they might even fear it...

And that one thing is...

Sucking on his penis after he's ejaculated!

Trust me, we have all been there – and very few men will tell you that the level of sensitivity is way too high after he's cum, and have that pressed between your lips is almost PAINFUL for him and is a sure-fire way to turn him off for your next session.

I've only ever known a couple men to openly admit that this feeling isn't nice. But, after chatting with an ex of mine, it's become pretty obvious that almost ALL men absolutely hate this.

And that includes yanking on it afterwards...

How to avoid this turn off: After you've made him cum, leave it alone. Make sure you are still stimulating his penis AS he cums with either your mouth or hand. But afterwards, just leave it alone and leave him to mop up on aisle one!

Turn off number two – Sex with a dead llama

Pardon the very disturbing image there...

But image how fun it would be to have sex...with a dead llama...

Would it be fun?

No, of course not.

My point here is that men get turned off by BORING sex. Really, if you want to keep your man in your bed, then you've got to liven your sex up – or at least keep it mildly entertaining for him.

Whilst you may love the thought of just lying there as he groans away on top of you, it won't be enough for a lot of men. Sex is very important when it comes to relationships and dating. Basically, a man wants to see how fun you are in bed before he commits to being with you – and the more fun you are in bed, the more likely you will get to keep him.

The turn off comes from not being 'adventurous' enough.

And trust me, a LOT of women fret over this issue – but really, it's simple enough to avoid.

How to avoid this turn off: You have to bear in mind that making love is something that we share between the two of us – not something where your main purpose is to enjoy YOURself. If you aim to pleasure HIM, then you will receive your reward in due course, and at the same time you will be satisfying his needs; not just yours.

This is going to sound a little weird – but hear me. Try watching some porn. I'm serious – give it a go. Even if it goes against whatever you believe in; no one will know but you, and you will get some great ideas from it.

That's not to say you have find the dirtiest hardcore porn on the internet, which is going to end up making you think the best way to please your man involves bananas and Vaseline...

Try searching for something slightly more 'sensual' and take note of how the 'female lead' acts and treats the man. Trust me; you will get some good ideas from this.

Turn off number three – That Vagina Thing...

Ok, we are all adults here (I hope), so let's get a talking about what men will probably never admit to getting turned off by – and that's the sound of your vagina farting. Whilst I hate to have to talk about such a topic, it's something that needs to be addressed because men DO get turned off by this, and for women, it can be a very embarrassing issue.

First off – if a guy leaves you because of this reason, then he's a DICK and you are better off without someone so lame. That's the truth.

Anyway, vaginal farts are causing by air entering your vagina, which is ultimately pushed in from his penis as you have sex. Unfortunately, this happens to every one of us and there is no definite 'cure' to the problem. However...

Since the problem revolves around air entering your vagina through sex, the best way to prevent the noise from happening, is by having your partner constantly inside you. This isn't actually as hard as it sounds. When you switch positions, try to naturally have him stay inside you, unless of course you are moving to a position where it's impossible. This will stop him from pushing all that damn air inside you. Think of his penis as some type of 'cork'.

Either that or you request that he doesn't pull the entire way out of you, thus not allowing air to enter. Don't be shy to talk to him about this and make such requests. He won't want to hear that noise just as much as you don't!

Sometimes the problem comes from different sexual positions. You SHOULD be able to notice which ones are making your vagina feel different, like air is entering. If not, then usually 'doggy style' is the main culprit for causing these 'varts' (vaginal fart slang). If so, switch up positions and find the one YOU are most comfortable with!

Turn off number four – Weird things!

Ok, so there are SOME men out there that like some really crazy forms of sex. And if you meet that type of guy, then you will soon know that they like that type of thing.

However, your average guy DOESN'T like weird forms of sex. Whilst its great fun to have adventurous sex, there is a line that most people won't cross, and if you try to force a guy to unexpectedly cross that line, he's gonna get turned off pretty quickly.

If you are interested in trying something different with your partner, then you should make sure that you discuss it with them FIRST instead of just trying it. And by those 'weird' type of things, I mean things like:

- Anal fingering. Sure, some guys like it - but a LOAD don't. You're going to want to ask him first before doing this.
- Toilet time – Oh God, this goes without saying, but before you decide to piss on your man's face or take a dump on his chest, why not talk to him first? There is a chance he will like the idea – but very unlikely. As in sure you don't like it either...
- Biting – ok some gentle 'biting' can be nice, but it's going to really hurt a guys most sensitive region if you decide to bite down on it with any substantial force
- Spitting – can be a turn on if you spit on his penis, but anywhere else, especially his face, is a big no no.

As I've said, if you want to try something that is considered 'different' then make sure you talk about it first to ensure that you are BOTH interested in trying it.

How to avoid this turn off: If you're having sex for the first time with your new guy, then keep it at a reasonable level of 'dirtiness' – if you talk to him, in time, you will find out what 'other things' he's into. Just make sure you don't surprise him with anything too 'different' or he might not want to come back for more...

Turn off number five – Insecurity

Join the club of the millions of other women who are insecure about their body. While it sucks to hate yourself, it sucks even more to try and hide yourself away during sex. When a man is horny enough, he isn't going to care about that spare tire you've got going, or that tiny spot on your inner thigh.

Trying to cover up your 'insecurities' is going to make your sex become stale. You're going to worry so much that you won't truly get into a sexual mood and enjoy a special experience with your partner.

Worrying about your insecurities WILL show, and your man will see it. For the most part he won't comment, but it may take him out of the 'mood' to the point where he doesn't see fit to have sex with you – or the sex just becomes boring.

How to avoid this turn off: I'd love to be able to tell you to just LOVE YOURSELF no matter what and have done with it – but we all know that it's never that easy.

If you feel you are carrying an extra bit of weight, and you really don't like having that on display, then you may want to go with having the majority of your sex lying on your back. Doing this will make you look slimmer and sexier, whilst keeping your belly tucked safely away.

I know, this sounds like a horrible solution, and you should be free to do whatever you like during sex – but for some people, extra weight can kill ALL self-esteem. Wearing a t-shirt during sex may be a short term solution, but if you are really concerned, then it's time to switch up your diet and join the gym. Joining the gym will change your life – I promise.

But at the end of the day, you are most likely having sex with someone who either likes you or LOVES you – and if they truly feel either way, then they won't be bothered by any of your 'insecurities' – in fact, they may even learn to love them!

Turn off number Six – Never making the first move

This pisses a lot of men off – and gets to the point where it's just downright frustrating.

A girl who NEVER makes the first move toward having sex is a major turn off – and it sucks badly.

Guys will have sex pretty much every night – but they don't want to HAVE to be the one to initiate sexual actions with you.

The problem will eventually lie within the guy's self-esteem. He's going to be sat there every night thinking 'why doesn't she want to?' – which of course makes a guys feel like he's not worthy enough to be approached for sex and becomes more of a mission to get you to want it.

If you're in the mood for sex, or even slightly so – then just go ahead and make a move on him. Just do it! He's very unlikely to turn you away.

Don't make having sex with your man a mission. It's not hard to lean over him and lay your lips on his to let him know you're in the mood. He will most likely take it from there. But not making any sort of move is so demoralising for men.

And acting like this, like it's a given for a man to initiate sex with you, makes you come across very BORING.

How to avoid this turn off: Don't be boring and expect your man to come to you when you need it. He has no idea when you are in the mood.

BONUS SECTION – What you wear

Ok, I wanted to include this in the 'in bed' section since it's too do with physical attraction, but it didn't seem like quite the right place to put it – so I've gone with a bonus section here on what things turn men on and off when it comes to clothing.

And yes, what you wear will have a massive effect on how your guy see's you in terms of turn ons and turn offs! Let's take a look first at what type of clothing turns men off.

Turns men off

Too much make-up – While you may want to make that extra effort to try and conceal every single last imperfection on your face, it just isn't worth it. Unless you have bad acne, people WON'T notice the small imperfections you behold, and covering them up with a tonne of make-up is going to make you look like a bloated clown.

Excessive cleavage – Wearing any item of clothing that reveals WAY too much cleavage is a terrible idea. The worst part here is that it makes a girl look SLUTTY and while some guys may desire sluts, it's not the type of attraction you want to gain. Plus, you want men primarily to be attracted your facial features – and having your tits riding out on your feet is going to be a massive distraction.

High riding thong – Again, it's taking all the attraction away from your facial features and makes you look like a slut. Whilst that may not be your intention, men will only be looking at your with sexual desires and nothing more. There is nothing wrong with wearing a thong, just make sure it isn't overly high when you are out and about.

Dressing like a celebrity – Seems like a good idea to copy popular people right? Wrong! Dressing the way celebs do makes you look like you don't have your own personality and makes you seem like an attention-whore. Some men won't know the difference, but the ones with any class will be able to see through the act.

General slutty clothes – Anything that makes you look like you charge $5 an hour is going to be a huge turn off for respectable men. You might think it's a good idea to show some skin, which it is – but showing too much is not nice.

Turns men on

When it comes to turning men on with your clothing, then you want to get the balance between sexual turn on and mental turn on just RIGHT – otherwise you are either going to come across as a whore or a library attendant.

Cleavage – Ok, when you are out for the night and you're looking to impress, feel free to show a BIT of cleavage. Not so much that the attention is taken away from your face - but just enough so that guys try and sneak a few peaks at what you got.

Of course, you don't need to show any cleavage to turn men on mentally and sexually, but it does help with attraction without making you look slutty. Some women refuse to show any skin whatsoever when they go out, and it often leads to men thinking that they are hiding something or just plain shy.

Skinny jeans – Tight jeans that reveal a nice figure are always a turn on for men, without making you look at all dirty. A nice fitting pair of jeans can highlight your awesome butt, if you have one – and go well with other clothes.

Men want to see some curves on a lady. Whilst there is nothing wrong with wearing baggy clothing (it is comfy), it just isn't a great way to impress men.

The color red – We associate red with a TONNE of emotional things in life – such as love, romance and sex.

Wearing red has been PROVEN to attract a lot more attention than any other color. So when you pick out your clothes for your next night out or date, it's a good idea to try and include SOME red. That doesn't mean you should go out looking like Santa Claus, though.

Backless clothes – Tops with the back revealing your beautiful spinal region are a HUGE turn on for guys. The lovely curve of a females back leaves loads to the imagination and can even look very classy when warn correctly.

Heals – Heals are sexy and classy, no matter what you wear them with – and men love a lady in heals. If you can wear heals and walk confidently, you are onto an instant winner. However, if you need practice walking in them, do so or make yourself look like a tit and ruin everything.

How you carry yourself – No matter what clothes you wear, it doesn't matter unless you know how to 'carry' yourself. I by 'carry yourself', I mean wearing the correct clothes for your physique.

We are ALL different, and not all of us are going to look good in skinny jeans. Take some time to find out what makes YOU look confident. And here's a tip for you: DON'T ask your female friends, they will most likely tell you that you look good in anything you wear...They are friends; they won't want to say anything bad, in general.

A better move, that I've always found, is to ask my father or brother. Men are much more brutal with their analysis, especially when it comes to family members. If father or brother isn't an option for you, then you may want to find a gay best friend – those guys know their shit!

What a lot of it boils down to, is how CONFIDENT you feel wearing your outfit. If you can go out feeling confident and not look overly slutty, you are a winner. Confidence is HOT.

IMAGINATION – A guys mind is his worst enemy when it comes to being turned on- and leaving as much as you can to the imagination will drive him WILD – trust me! Always give a sample of what you have to offer, but never give him the full package UNLESS he's earned it over time.

MEGA-AWESOME QUICK LIST OF OTHER TURN OFFS!

- Having facial hair! Shave or bleach that shit ladies!
- Unibrow – two brows are better than one!
- THAT bush – a little hair 'down there' is fine – but keep it trimmed - ideally! Men love a well groomed female.
- A good smelling vagina. I needed say more.
- Teethy BJS – use your LIPS not your TEETH when sucking.
- Farting. Don't do it unless you are in a 70 year old relationship.
- Crying too much. Hopefully not during sex!
- Messy hair.
- Faking 'it' 'UHHHH OHHHH YEAAAH BABY UUOOORRGHHH'
- Being over-theatrical.
- NOT MENTIONING YOUR PERIOD. Even worse when sexing...
- General selfishness. Share the love in and out of bed.
- Granny underwear.
- Excessive drunk behaviour. Control your drinking if you want to impress men.
- Trying to give too many directions when having sex..
- Telling a man how he should dress.
- Boring conversation. *'How was your day?'* Yaaaawn.
- Texting while in his company. Phones away.
- Dirty faces. If you need to do them, practice in a mirror or you most likely look like a possum sucking a lemon.
- Dirty underwear.

Okidoke then – let us move on once again to the next part of my lovely book, yeh?

How to Become His PERFECT Fantasy Girl

Here's what you're about to learn inside (get excited NOW):

- How to become a sex GODDESS without being 'slutty' or 'weird'

- How to IGNITE his emotions without even laying a finger on him

- Exciting bed tips that will leave him BREATHLESS

- Sexy games to spice up your love life FAST

Ok, so I don't want to drag on and keep you waiting. I tend to write my books with no BS so you can get straight to the goods.

Let's do this.

First things first – WHY you need to be a naughty girl

Let's get one thing straight: being a NAUGHTY girl, doesn't mean you have to be a slutty girl. In fact, respectable men are actually TURNED OFF by women who are overly whore-like.

A naughty girl is one who is able to tease, create erotic tension and excitement without having to resort straight to sexual activities.

But if you're in a relationship, why is it so important to act naughty?

Well, simple: because it's exciting. People want to commit to relationships because they are very exciting, sexually and mentally. For years now, men and women have been cheating on their partners for one reason; and that's because the relationship isn't EXCITING enough.

Acting slutty is for women who just want to hop straight into bed to sort their own needs out. The 'naughty girl' drives her man wild with erotic excitement before he's even had the chance to undress her.

Here's a summary of why you NEED to become that naughty girl:

- Create excitement in the relationship

- Keep your man thinking of you

- Make him HORNY in public

- Enjoy sex more

- Make him want you every night, even though he can't

- Create a FIREY bond between the two of you

- Become his FANTASY GIRL

- You break out of the 'normal' type of girl stereotype

Men LOVE this. They want a sweet girlfriend who knows how to tease them and make them earn your pussy. Anything that is handed to a man on a plate is going to get eaten up like bacon and never truly respected.

Grab yourself a strong drink, brace yourselves and get ready to learn how to become his FANTASY GIRL.

Note: In all my books, I teach women how to become DESIREABLE whilst keeping their respect and dignity intact, without having to resort to slutty measures.

If you are looking for masturbation techniques that will have your man shooting across States, then you've come to the wrong place.

What is considered 'Slutty'?

I get asked this question a lot. And there is definitely a difference between being slutty and being naughty.

Being slutty suggested you have no boundaries and is often a word associated with women who sleep with multiple men – which if you are in a relationship, I will assume you aren't doing that.

Here are a few bullet points to help you understand what I consider 'slutty' and won't be covering in this book. Bear in mind, I keep these out of the equation in order to keep that respectable yet naughty balance just perfect:

- Sending nude pictures of yourself (once sent, it's out of your control)

- Sleeping with multiple men

- Dressing like a whore in everyday situations

- Having nothing but sexual chats on phone/text

- Giving him sex whenever he wants it (doesn't make you a slut but it doesn't make you the 'naughty' girl we want either)

Again, to reiterate my point: this book is about becoming an EXTREMELY sexually desirable person whilst keep respectable boundaries between you and your man.

And whilst we are here, those 'weird' sexual acts that you may have seen on the internet don't make you a naughty girl, they make you a weird girl. Sure, some people will into that type of shit, but most people AREN'T. Experimenting in bed is great fun, but you need to know when your naughty act is becoming a slightly 'weird' act.

For example:

- Trying to finger your man without permission

- Having an array of bondage gear laid out on your bed ready

- Pissing on your man

- Shitting on your man

- Having your neighbour hide in the cupboard then jump out naked mid-sex to surprise your man.

Again, some people like this stuff – and if you do, that's totally cool. But you need to check with your man prior to attempting things like it before initiating them.

Being a respectable and sweet girl with a naughty mind, who knows how to use it the right way is where YOU want to be.

Here's the first and most important step – CHANGE

So, you want to drive your man wild - but you don't know how to, yet.

Chances are, that your idea of being his 'fantasy woman' involve dressing up in sexy lingerie and having humplings for breakfast, lunch and dinner – which is fine, but it's not the way of a true naughty girl.

But if you want to become a TRUE sexy, boner-inducing GODESS then you most likely need to CHANGE the way you are acting sexually with your man – and this means IN and OUT of bed.

Here's what you need to change FIRST:

Giving him his sex when HE wants

This is most likely your first mistake; giving him sex whenever HE wants to have it. The true raw emotional urge for sex comes from NOT letting him have it, or even better; making him EARN the sex.

It's true; a man wants what he can't have. That's not to say you have to deprive the poor soul of his sexy-time - in fact, that's probably going to get him worried. By using the sexy mind games throughout this book, in tandem with the correct timing of using them, you will have your man driven WILD in no time.

But, in the mean time, he has to wait for YOU to be the one to initiate sex with him. Not only does the wait drive his ass crazy, but when he finally feels he's earned the pleasure of being able to have you; he will ravish you like never before - and you will LOVE it as much as him.

So when should I let him have it?

Of course, you shouldn't be the one to initiate sexual activity with your partner EVERY time - but if you wanna make your man's nuts go nuts, then you need to know when to reward him. By getting him hornier than he's ever been before, then letting him get between your legs is a TRUE reward for your man.

Half of the fun comes from the ANTICIPATION and build up, and the other half, the actual sex.

So, in this book, I will break down your naughty girl activity into TWO sections: minds games, and physical games. And after each 'technique' I will guide you to EXACTLY how you should perform the technique and how long you should make your man wait before letting him have at you (if at all).

So - this is it, this is where the fun behinds ladies!

Mind games - What and why?

Mind games are the penultimate sexual pleasure; THE best way to drive your man wild without physical touch. And as previously stated; half the fun comes from the build up toward sex, and mind games are PERFECT for doing this - if you know how to!

Mind games are the little things you can do throughout the day to get your man into a crazy sexual mood. Naughty girl mind games are not to be mistaken for childish mind games. And as I teach in ALL my books, these type of mind games AREN'T nice, i.e., trying to make someone overly jealous to want you more.

So, without further ado, let's take a look at the TOP minds games you can play with your man, and when you need to do them.

Mind game number one – Sexting

SEXTING, as much as it paints me to say it; but it's real, and it's a totally awesome way to get your guy in the mood - if you know how of course.

Sexting, in case you didn't know, is the slang term for sexual texting (sending sexual text messages) and should ONLY be used if you are already in a committed relationship, which I assume, if you are reading this, which you are.

When performed correctly, sexting can be a powerful game. But, what is your idea of sexting? And how often should you do it?

What effective sexting ISN'T:

- Overly graphic descriptions of sexual acts

- Sending NUDE pictures

- Engaging in sexting when HE wants

Obviously this type of communication between partners should be kept confidential, but the amount of times I've heard about women attempting to sext their other half's and FAILING is unreal - and it's mostly down to these three points.

First off, let's talk about sending nude pictures of yourself. Sure, it's going to get your man hot under the collar - but is it really worth it? Remember, that once you send a picture of yourself like that to someone, you may NEVER get it back - and what they do with that picture down the road, you can never be sure of.

Generally, feel free to stay away from sending ANY pictures of yourself in order to tease. More on that shortly.

This brings me on to...

'MMM BABE CAN'T WAIT TO SUCK YOUR JUICY LOVE STICK TONIGHT'

While that may create a mass of brief excitement for your man, knowing he's going to get sex that evening, it doesn't have that true NAUGHTY GIRL factor that we're looking for.

SECRET SAUCE: NEVER tell him what he going to get. Let his mind become his own worst enemy. The real fun from sexting comes from SUGGESTIVE texts throughout the day that make him horny but don't reveal or not he's actually going to get his little treat in bed.

And if he tries to be the one to initiate a real dirty sexual conversation with you, then it's your duty to TAKE the power away from him sit yourself directly in the driver's seats. Here's an example:

 Him - 'Let's fuck tonight. I wanna do so much to you babe...'

You - 'Great to hear! ;)'

No matter what; there is NO need to get into graphic sexual texts. Do your best to keep your man's mind thinking. Sexting is NOT the exchange of dirty texts, not for us anyway.

DO NOT send nude pictures

DO NOT tell him what he wants to hear

DO NOT organise sexual activities with him

DO NOT allow him to control your sexting conversation

So that's told us what sexting isn't, now let's look at what it is and how to drive your man wild.

How to sext him wild

- Create anticipation and excitement

- Make suggestively sexual messages

- Take control of his emotions when YOU want

So, this section is a little difficult, as sexting is something that you really need to practice to become perfect at - SO, I figured it would be a good idea if I just go ahead and SHOW you my top favourite tease text messages that I've used in the past.

Obviously you won't want to keep using the same ones over and over - but this will help you get an idea of how to create those exciting mildly sexual and suggestive messages.

First off, let's take a look at how your sexts need to be structured. Here's a basic guideline for what to include into a seductive text.

EXCITE > INTRUIGE > TEASE > ENGAGE

Let's take a look at a few examples and why they work so well:

(Bearing in mind, here we will be the ones who initiate the sexting, not him)

Also, please be sure to use these texts at the CORRECT time, and how often you should do this to keep the excitement - which I will discuss shortly after these examples.

Oh one last thing: feel free to skip on formalities - just dive straight in, trust me.

SAUCY QUESTIONS

'What's the sexiest outfit you think I could wear?'

'Have you ever felt horny whilst texting me?'

'If you were here with me, what would you want to do to me?'

(When he texts back after this text, IGNORE his reply. He will think he hasn't done well enough and will try harder later to prove his worth)

'What's your idea of great foreplay?'

(Again, ignore his response)

Bear in mind: If he gets shitty with you for ignoring his texts, just tell him you were busy.

These are just a few examples of GREAT texts to send your man. Take a look at how they are structured. Not ONCE do I say anything sexual myself, but the tone is set as being very sexual indeed.

He knows we are talking dirty here, and he's also being challenged to impress you with his answers - which men LOVE to do. And of course, if you text these out of the blue, his intrigue levels will shoot through the roof.

Demands are great, especially when out of the blue. The put you in control and create an unusual like situation for any man. These texts break the 'usual' pattern and put you firmly in control whilst turning him on.

SAUCY DEMANDS

'You should wear those ripped jeans tonight. You look sexy in them! Shame you will have to keep them on though! ;) '

Plenty of demands you can come up with! You shouldn't need me here...

How often and when should I use such sexts?

As with most things in life, repetitiveness becomes boring - and the same goes for sexting. If you text the same things to your man every day, the act will start to wear thin and the effectiveness will become less.

In order to keep things exciting, it's imperative that you come up with variations of the texts above. Like I said, practice will make perfect! To make sure you keep your man excited, don't stick with a 'pattern' or he will know when to expect the fun.

Try this monthly pattern to begin with:

Week 1 - Just one text

Week 2 - Three sexts a week

Week 3 - Two sexts a week

Week 4 - Inundate him with sexts

Week 5 (start of next month) - NO sexts

This is the exact plan I used to drive my man absolutely insane with horniness. And the beautiful part of this comes from week 5, the NO SEXT week.

NO SEXT week breaks the pattern, intrigues him, drives him wild and let's him know what life is like without you getting him worked. Just make sure you don't go too long without texting him SOMETHING sexually suggestive; it makes a guy think something is up. Just make sure you get back into things the second week of that month.

Now, some of you may be thinking 'this seems like a lot of work to please a man' – but trust me, it's not. Even the smallest of suggestive sexts can wreak havoc on a guy's mind (in a good way). Even if you sent just one small sext a week, you can still keep your man guessing and on edge throughout the day – TRUST ME!!!

Your current situation

I understand that each person reading this book will be in a different 'position' with their love life. While this book is aimed at people who are in adult, committed relationships, that doesn't mean the techniques won't work for people who are just casually dating, because they will!

If you are casually dating, then these sexts are AWESOME – but you need to make sure you have at least developed some kind of 'relationship' with the person you are involved with, in the sense that you should have known them, and been talking to them, for some time (and preferably sexually active with). Otherwise, you're going to come across as a slut, basically.

And as for those of you in committed relationships; some of you may be living together; some of you may not be living together. Ideally, this book is aimed at those of you who AREN'T living together, because it gives you that time alone to create the excitement of when you next meet up.

If you ARE living together, my suggestion would be that you SERIOUSLY monitor the time that you spend together, and work out a way that allows you both to get excited about having free time together, thus allowing you to incorporate these SEXTS. A classic way of doing this is to text your man whilst he's at work; let him read your sexts when he's on his break or on his way home – works a treat!

Mind game number two – No touching

Yes, we all know already that you don't need to touch a man to drive his sexual desires into overdrive – but many of us don't know HOW to do this.

As we already know, a man's worst enemy is his own mind. And allowing him to manifest our slight sexual suggestions into overwhelming sexual fantasies can be achieved VERY easily. Let's take a look at some of the TOP ways to turn him on without engaging in any physical touching.

What you wear

A lot of the time, this turn on happens naturally – but you should want to harness the true power of this by being able to turn him on with what you wear, whenever YOU want.

The key here is to, as usual, leave something to his imagination – and my favourite way to do this is by showing just a **little bit of bra strap**, purposely just slightly moved to one side of my shoulder blade.

Don't ask me why, but this can drive a guy nuts. Maybe it's the thought of being able to see something that he shouldn't be able to see unless you are engaged in sexual activity. This is a great way to play with his mind when out in public.

Next I'd recommend wearing something with a **TIGHT FIT**, showing off the curves of your body. That doesn't mean you have to wear LESS clothes, just ones that compliment your figure better.

Showing off **the small of your back**; for a lot of men, this is an absolutely HUGE turn on – and as with all my techniques, it makes you look sexy without having to look 'slutty'

There are of course a TONNE of sexy clothes you can wear to impress your man, but generally, when it comes to toying around in public, these are the TOP ways to get him hot under the collar without attracting too much unwanted attention.

How often should I dress like it?

It's gonna make you look slightly stupid if you prance around with a crooked bra strap every time you go out with your man. To avoid looking like a woman who can't dress herself and come across as one who knows how to tease, you should of course limit the amount of times you do this.

For me, I use these techniques very rarely – and I find that's what works best between me and my man. This way, he doesn't know what to expect and when to expect it. Seriously, just a few times a month in a variety of different scenarios will do the trick. The goal here isn't to have him ripping your clothes off in public, but to slowly build sexual tension, along with the other techniques in the book.

TURN ON LEVEL: TWO STARS

Something a little hotter now – The Peep Show

This is a method I use to really drive my man wild – and it works like mad. And I like to call this one, 'The peep show'.

I call it The peep show for obvious reasons. What we will be doing here, is letting our man take a look at what he's not going to get. And not letting him have what he sees is a vital part of the overall turn on.

All you need to do is let your man WATCH you as you either undress, or take a shower. It's a lot of guys' fantasies to be able to watch someone undress or take a shower, so even if you don't let him get the goods afterwards, he will still be hugely turned on.

The following sentence is all you need to get started:

'I want you to watch me undress/take a shower for the next 10 minutes'

It's a powerful sentence, as not only does it intrigue and EXCITE – but it also gives the impression that you're going to let him have sex with you, even though you won't – just yet.

After you've finished dressing or having a shower, he will most likely try to make a move on you. And this is exactly the point where you keep him waiting by telling him 'not tonight, but soon'.

At this point you may be thinking 'When they hell do I let him have my sexy time?' – And that's perfectly fine. In the second half of the book we will be going through a tonne of very HOT sexual moves and plays for you and your man to get on with.

But in order for him to perform at his highest potential with these sexual plays, you need to go through the mind games section first and build his horniness levels up as high as possible. Trust me!

How often should I?

For me, this worked best using it VERY rarely. Once a month was absolutely perfect. He eventually knew his little peep show treat was going to come each month, but I'd never let him know for sure.

TURN ON LEVEL: 4 STARS

Mind game number three – Exercise

I'm going to try and keep this chapter short, since it's pretty simple technique.

Exercising in front of your man is a killer way to get his imagination going.

I'm pretty sure that every guy has that fantasy of being alone in a yoga class with a beautiful woman in tight pants, who for some reason finds him desirable enough to bang him right then and there on the floor...

If you're living together, then perfect. Get a yoga mat out and put on a yoga DVD, dress up in tight-ass clothes and strut your stuff in front of him.

If you're not living together, then what I suggest is that you both hit the gym, at the same time. Not only will the sight of you bending over and sweating turn him on – but the natural effect exercise has on him with ENHANGE the horniness even more.

How often? For me, this comes on a whim; just do it whenever you feel like exercising. The beauty here is that he will be absolutely clueless that you are trying to tease him into a horny state, whilst looking oh so innocent in the process.

TURN ON LEVEL: 2.5 STARS

QUICK FIRE ROUND

Here's an ultra quick fire round of other ways you can turn your man on without physical contact:

Confidence – Oh yeah, confidence is hot! Men love a woman who is in control of her actions. Even if you don't feel confident, it's so easy to look it – stand tall, keep your hair off your face, speak slowly and ACT like a confident person. Take a look at people you consider to be confident and COPY them – and in time, natural confidence will come.

Smile – A big warm smile can surprisingly cause a big warm smile in man's pants too. Keep your teeth looking good, and just smile baby.

Compliment – Treat your man to the occasional compliment about his physical attributes. Don't inundate him with compliments, just pick a few out of the blue about his muscles arms or big shoulders and he will love you for it.

(This is one of the few occasions where it's OK to maybe lie just a little)

Perfume – Ok, I should have made a separate section for this, maybe – but the right perfume alone can get a guy HARD. Trust me, spending that extra few dollars on the perfect scent is absolutely vital for getting your man worked up.

Eye contact – When talking to your man, hold an extra long gaze during silent parts of your conversation. Your deep stare will do the talking for you. Remember to throw in a small smile or you're gonna look like a serial killer.

Red – When picking out ANY outfit, make extra efforts to wear SOME visible red. Red promotes sexual emotions from men subconsciously – so wear it!

LISTEN UP!

Now, this is where the REAL naughty girl fun happens. In the bed!

With the combination of the mind game techniques above, put together should be able to drive your man into a horny overdrive. Now's the time to let him have it.

But when exactly?

Men get horny at anything. Just the sight of a pair of boobs is enough to get them horny. Getting them to have sex with us isn't the problem. Getting them to perform like an animal that wants to please a sexy goddess however, is!

The temptation will be to let him have sex with you even after you've just used a few of these techniques – and that's fine, if you want. But to take things to the next level, you HAVE to tease him into it and make him EARN it.

That's not to say you have to deprive your man of sex, oh no – God forbid! But giving it to him whenever he wants it is not the way forward. As with most techniques in this book, the general rule of thumb is: **BE UNPREDICTABLE**.

You might call me crazy, but I started to limit the amount of times I had sex with my man to less than ONCE A WEEK. *burn her!*

The reason being; regular sex can become pretty stale after being in a committed relationship for a while. I've stuck with these same rules and methods and have been in some extremely exciting and rewarding relationships. I am now still using these techniques to keep things with my current man fresh and exciting. But hey, what do I know; we've only been together for 15 years. ☺

Enough about me; let's get naughty.

SEX GAMES

Now, you've probably heard about spicing things up with 'sex games' before, but what you haven't heard; is WHICH games are guaranteed to drive your man crazy with pleasure. Let's take a look at the best ones.

Gone in 60 seconds

Simple, fast and adrenaline fuelled. Gone in 60 seconds is a game you can play with you man that puts the pressure and focus ENTIRELY on him, and it's crazy exciting for him. Here's how it's done.

Aim of the game: The aim of the game is to CHALLENGE your man to cum whilst you watch him. He's not allowed to touch you and has to pleasure himself ONLY. You can make this a team effort by posing in sexy positions and pulling cute faces.

If he wins: If he can achieve this, then you have to let him fulfil a sexual fantasy of him the next time you have some bed fun.

If he loses: Put the thought of not allowing him to have sex with you for 2 weeks if he doesn't cum within 60 seconds. Of course, you don't need to torture the poor fella if he doesn't manage. The fear adds to the adrenaline!

Not tonight...Maybe

Not tonight, maybe – is my absolute FAVOURITE sex game to play. And you got to be careful with this one; it can drive both of you mad with sexual rage (the good kind).

Aim of the game: The aim of the game here is to get into bed with your man, in your sexiest outfit, engage in lots of foreplay – and try your best NOT to have penetrative sex. The levels of arousal this can cause are THROUGH THE ROOF.

Engage in as much kissing, touching, caressing and teasing as you can – eventually one of you will take the step toward sex. Don't be cruel and leave your man blue-balled!

If he wins: If you're the one who takes the step toward penetrative sex, then it's your night to take control of him. Ride him, grind him, and make him feel like his cock is king for the night. That's his prize.

If he loses: And starts having full on sex with you, then that's your treat to be able to just lie there and let him make ALL the effort that night. Bad boy.

The Alpha Male

As we already know; men LOVE to be in control of most situations. And the typical man likes to feel like the alpha male in all walks of life. So, with this next game, it's time to let your man be The Alpha Male.

Aim of the game: This one's a little tricky to set up – but the reward is totally awesome. Throughout the day, it's your job to do things that you know WIND your man up, not in a sexual way, but in a general frustration way.

This should be mostly irrelevant things, as they will just be used as reference later on during the game. Small things like forgetting to pick something up from the grocery store. Try and get about ten mistakes into one day.

Once you get into bed with your partner, it's time to allow him to release his vented frustration. Sit him up on the bed and tell him you were purposely trying to piss him off today, and now you think it's time for him to punish you.

Pull down your pants, bend over the bed and demand that he gives you 60 seconds worth of spanking for every mistake you've made that day.

There is no winner and loser in this game. But usually, this ends with very rough sex – so be prepared and in the mood if you choose to go this route.

Plain old role-play

Some guys are waaay too shy to ever admit it, but they most likely LOVE role-playing, and it's actually easier to do than you may think.

First off, there are a few types of 'roles' that hit home best and they may not be what you were expecting. Here's what the best ones are:

Cheerleader – Goes without saying really. Pretty much every guy loves a cute girl in a short skirt outfit acting all cute and shit...

Police officer – Yep, if you can get a hold of the gear, it's a huge turn on for your man – and can go great with a night of dominating him.

Prostitute – Unbelievable but true. A lot of guys have that fantasy of hooking up with a complete stranger for organised sex. Fortunately, most have the decency not to go through with it, but this gives him that little chance to give it a go.

That's All Folks

Thank you for taking the time to read my little report! I appreciate it.

And I would really appreciate it if you followed the advice in this guide. You will have more success that you think! Trust me!

Please stay tuned for other HOT reports soon...

Thank you!

Melanie Raymund